Real Fibromyalgia Rx

Fibromyalgia, Chronic Fatigue Syndrome, and Interstitial Cystitis – A Pituitary Perspective

Acknowledgments

This book could not have been written without a lot of good people who've suffered, putting their faith in me as a physician. None of this could have been accomplished without the leadership and incredible knowledge of Nabil Gemayel, MD, probably the best and nicest pituitary endocrinologist in the United States. He's also a cardiologist. Many patients now live fuller and more normal lives because of him. The work of Troy Lund, MD was key to helping this work come together – God bless him. I'd like to give a big thanks to Dr. Steven Freestone (MD Pathologist) of the Utah Valley Regional Medical Center in Provo, Utah. He was always available to answer even the most ridiculous questions regarding lab techniques and levels. Thanks to Kimball Crofts, MD, a kind and talented plastic surgeon, for allowing some of this work to move forward in his beautiful office space. Michael Jensen, MD, started all this years ago. He is one of the kindest physicians I know. Richard Rosenthal, MD, of the Nexus Pain Clinic tolerated our endless discussions of the chicken or the egg theory on pain. And I cannot forget Neal Rouzier, MD., of Clinics of the Palm Deserts in Palm Springs. He is a hormone doctor who has taught so many physicians, and is years ahead of everyone else. Thank you Neal – this work is for you too.

Also, thanks to the patients and the staff of Aesthetica Preventive Medicine Institute LLC, where a lot of this work was done and ideas proved – especially Denise, Brenna and Caroline – you rock!

Thank you to the awesome physicians and staff of the Clinica Medica Familiar in Santa Ana, California for their long-suffering assistance in our research there. We would randomly appear to take over their exam rooms, and they never complained. They are humble and kind practitioners of the healing arts.

I owe thanks to two key pharmacies. First, thanks to MedQuest® Pharmacy in Utah (www.mqrx.com). They have been a leader in compounding for decades. They make some of the best hormone products on the planet. Also, thanks to Nayan Patel PhD and his team at Central Drug® in La Habra, California. This is the most excellent group of compounding and pharmaceutical geniuses I know. Nayan is a lecturer at the University of Southern California – a skill in which he excels. Dr. Gemayel is a talented lecturer as well. The work could not have moved forward without their long hours of dedicated service.

There are many people who allowed this work to move forward, too many to list. Thanks to you all.

Foreword

After a long day seeing patients and doing testing, I was sitting with Dr. Nabil Gemayel in a hamburger joint in downtown Santa Ana, California. I asked him what he thought of fibromyalgia. Without a pause he replied, "It's pituitary damage that's undiagnosed – it's a growth hormone deficiency."

I felt shocked by his answer. I looked at him and asked, "Really?"

"Yes, absolutely" he said and went back to his fries.

I took his answer seriously. This brilliant man had trained at Harvard in pituitary endocrinology, had worked at the NIH and Walter Reed for a couple of decades, and then had been named assistant to the US Surgeon General. He was at USC only *after* he'd completed a cardiology fellowship. He's a cardiologist *and* a pituitary endocrinologist. He was one of the pre-eminent physicians on the west coast – I'd *better* take it seriously.

That's how this book began, in a hamburger joint in Santa Ana, California.

This book is not earth-shattering – most of my information I obtained from the excellent modern medical literature that already exists, much like in my Program120® book on proactive preventive medicine. I hope that what I have written here and what I have presented in my educational endeavors is solid data, backed by research and by my own clinical experience. Fibromyalgia syndrome (called a syndrome because no one seems to know the cause) is a mysterious disease process to most caregivers and to nearly all patients – it should not be. I hope to shed light on this problem. I want to clarify the diagnostic issues involved, and indicate proper therapy that can be applied when a patient is accurately diagnosed. This is "root cause medicine" (like I teach in my Program120® lectures and textbook) and is exacting in its scope. Fibromyalgia cannot be "cured," but with careful skill and caring, the symptoms can be mostly resolved. Patients can go forward and live a nearly normal life.

My approach is not new – hypothalamic-pituitary-axis (HPA) problems and issues have been scrutinized as an etiology for fibromyalgia, but I try to connect those dots with a little different eye and experience. Don't think I'm being critical -- there are many really good, kind, caring professionals trying to do the right thing. The root causes of pituitary dysfunction or damage are multi-factorial, which adds to the immense confusion I see in this area. I'll try to explain all of those causes. This will lead to clarification in the diagnosis and treatment of this syndrome.

In the following text I'll make my case.

~Dan Purser, MD

Chapter 1
Fibromyalgia; Theories and Opinions

Discovering the Meaning of Real Fibromyalgia: Problems with Big Medicine and Big Pharmaceutical Companies

Much of what physicians learn on the job and at so-called "educational" conferences comes from pharmaceutical companies. Don't get me wrong – I believe pharmaceutical companies have improved the modern world with incredible medications, but it is a lazy error by physicians to depend on self-serving pharmaceutical companies to be the sole source of their ongoing education. I remind doctors of the phrase *caveat emptor* – buyers beware. Or in this case, patient *and* physician beware. It's our responsibility to do our homework, not to rely on pharmaceutical representatives. It's the doctors' job to know what's going on. They shouldn't be too busy to figure it out, I believe that handing over our education to drug manufacturing entities, or to hospital chains who benefit from unnecessary surgical interventions, or even to insurance companies that benefit from the belief that no therapies work for these patients, undermines appropriate care of many kinds of patients, especially those with the "fibromyalgia syndrome."

I don't know what pressure will be brought to bear on me because of what I've written, but the literature I present and the therapies I suggest have been proved with numerous patients over many clinical years of experience. I also realize that "connecting of the dots" in this book is done via my clinical experiences at Program120®. You'll see throughout the text that I suggest larger long-term multi-center double-blind trials to further validate this data.

Some Caregivers' Opinions

To present all opinions on this complex matter, let's hear what physicians are saying. Here are some excerpts from an article by an excellent doctor in Utah named Hugo Rodier, MD. He's an expert in integrative medicine. His article was printed in the Utah Medical Association *UMA Bulletin,* Volume 52, Number 2 from February 2005, available at www.utahmed.org.

"It seems *the FDA feels their clients are really the pharmaceutical companies, not the American public, according to whistle-blower Dr. David Graham,* interviewed by the U.S. Senate and PBS's *Now* news program.

(www.pbs.org/now/transcript/transcriptNOW101_full.html)

"When a great profession and the forces of capitalism interact, drama is likely to result. This has certainly been the case where the profession of medicine and the pharmaceutical industry are concerned. *On display in the relationship between doctors and drug companies are the grandeur and weaknesses of the medical profession, its noble aspirations and its continuing inability to fulfill them. Also on display are the power, social contributions and occasional venality of a very profitable industry whose products contribute in important ways to the health and longevity of the American people but that at times employs methods that are deeply troubling and even criminal.* Government also plays a part as it tries with limited success to help the profession stay true to its own tenets and to deter the industry's most egregious excesses. The spectacle is profoundly human and like most such spectacles, seems never to end or to lose its fascination."

Doctors and drug companies, *NEJM*2004;351:1885

"Statins' benefits are largely independent of initial LDL and total cholesterol concentrations ... Statins reduce the risk of Myocardial infarction more than would be predicted from the reduction in cholesterol achieved."

"Statins and micronutrients: unanswered questions," is the editorial that accompanied the article on statins presented above. (*J. Lancet* 2004;97:459)

"Medical education should prepare students for the clinical problems they will face in their future practice. However, that is not happening for the most prevalent problem in health care today: chronic disease [which comprises] 78 percent of health expenditures.

"Chronic disease has dramatically transformed the role of the patient... [he/she] becomes experienced and is often more knowledgeable than the physician about the effects of the disease and its treatment, and has an integral role in the treatment process ... knowledgeable patients achieve a better outcome. A collaborative physician improves both understanding by patients and health outcomes ... Unfortunately *few if any medical schools are preparing their students adequately."*

I love that excerpt from **"Chronic disease: the need for a new clinical education,"** *JAMA*2004;292: 1057. It explains why most physicians fail to help people with chronic conditions while we do quite well with acute problems like emergency room visits, heart attacks, and trauma caused by car accidents.

[All the above italics were added by this author.]

There is no magic bullet to "cure" chronic disease. The process to help someone return to near normalcy is tedious and complex. I spend hours per week helping patients. I spend time evaluating them and holding their hands. It's almost always hugely beneficial for the suffering patient and for their family as they realize some return to normalcy is indeed possible.

Chapter 2
The Definition and History of Fibromyalgia

Modern Definition of Fibromyalgia

The National Library of Medicine has more than 10,000 articles related to fibromyalgia[1]. Researchers are trying to discover the cause of fibromyalgia syndrome. All of this data has added to the confusion and often muddies the waters.

Defining the disease symptoms and diagnostic criteria is arduous, as noted in various recent articles:

"To date, there is *no "gold standard" for diagnosing fibromyalgia.* Until a better clinical case definition of fibromyalgia exists, all diagnostic criteria should be interpreted with caution, considered rudimentary, and subject to modification[2]." *[Italics and bold added by this author.]*

Because there **are** *no specific laboratory tests* **for fibromyalgia**, the 1990 American College of Rheumatology (ACR) classification criteria have been used in clinical settings; however, they are not ideal for individual patient diagnosis. Clinicians should be aware of limitations inherent in using tender points in the diagnosis of fibromyalgia. The multiple symptoms of fibromyalgia often overlap with those of related disorders and may further complicate the diagnosis[3]." *[Italics and bold added by this author.]*

"There is *still no gold standard for making a diagnosis of fibromyalgia*, but there is an increasing consensus for the development of new guidelines for diagnosis that modifies the currently prescribed tender point evaluation[4]." *[Italics and bold added by this author.]*

Regardless of the ongoing clinical opinions and research, definitions are still attempted.

"Fibromyalgia is a common nonarticular **disorder of unknown cause** characterized by generalized aching (sometimes severe), widespread tenderness of muscles, areas around tendon insertions, and adjacent soft tissues, as well as muscle stiffness, fatigue and poor sleep. Diagnosis is clinical. Treatment includes exercise, local heat, stress management, drugs to improve sleep, and analgesics."

From *The Merck Manuals Online Medical Library*

"In fibromyalgia, any fibromuscular tissues may be involved, especially those of the occiput, neck, shoulders, thorax, low back, and thighs. There is no specific histologic abnormality. Symptoms and signs are generalized, in contrast to localized soft-tissue pain and tenderness (myofascial pain syndrome—see also <u>Temporomandibular Disorders: Myofascial Pain Syndrome</u>), which is often related to overuse or microtrauma.

Fibromyalgia is common; it is about **7 times more common among women**, usually young or middle-aged women, but can occur in men, children, and adolescents.

11

Because of the sex difference, it is sometimes overlooked in men. **It sometimes occurs in patients with systemic rheumatic disorders.**

The cause is unknown, but **disruption of stage 4 sleep may contribute,** as can emotional stress. Patients may tend to be perfectionists. Fibromyalgia **may be precipitated by a viral or other systemic infection (e.g. Lyme disease) or a traumatic event**[5]**."**

[The bold added by this author.]

This is a generally accepted definition of fibromyalgia but it's incomplete.

Look at these phrases again, because these will become more important as we go through the data we have:

1. It is a disorder of unknown cause.
2. It is seven times more common among women than men.
3. It sometimes occurs in patients with systemic rheumatic disorders.
4. Disruption of stage 4 sleep may contribute.
5. It may be *precipitated* by a viral or other systemic infection (eg, Lyme disease) or a traumatic event.

I'll explain through independent studies and articles how this definition is wrong, how these five simple points are critical, and how this disease is not of unknown cause, but from a very clearly defined cause. It is a disease whose symptoms have been long mistreated, when in reality it can and should be properly diagnosed and treated.

The History of Fibromyalgia Syndrome

"Although the term "fibromyalgia" was not coined until 1976, people throughout history have reported illnesses with strikingly similar symptoms. These reports can be found as far back as Old Testament Biblical times.

Early Evidence: *Job* vividly described his physical anguish: "I, too, have been assigned months of futility, long and weary nights of misery. When I go to bed, I think, 'When will it be morning?' But the night drags on, and I toss till dawn ... And now my heart is broken. Depression haunts my days. My weary nights are filled with pain as though something were relentlessly gnawing at my bones." (Job 7:3-4; 30:16-17 - New Living Translation™)

Another well-known person who reported fibromyalgia-like symptoms was *Florence Nightingale*, an English army nurse during the Crimean War (1854-1856) who was a pioneer in the International Red Cross movement. Nightingale became ill while working on the front lines and never really recovered. She was virtually bedridden much of the rest of her life, with pain and fatigue symptoms resembling fibromyalgia until her death in 1910.

Florence Nightingale (original photograph, 1856, Perry Special Collection).

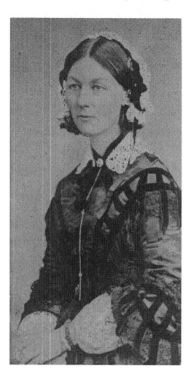

Terminology: This illness has been studied since the 1800s and has been identified by a variety of names; hysterical paroxysm, muscular rheumatism and fibrositis. The term fibromyalgia was coined in 1976 in an effort to describe its primary symptom. (Fibro – meaning fibrous tissue, my – meaning muscle, and algia – meaning pain).

It wasn't until 1990, when the American College of Rheumatology developed a diagnostic criteria for doing fibromyalgia research, that the term fibromyalgia gained wide usage.

1990 Criteria for the Classification of Fibromyalgia

1. History of widespread pain.

> *Definition.* Pain is considered widespread when all of the following are present: pain in the left side of the body, pain in the right side of the body, pain above the waist, and pain below the waist. In addition, axial skeletal pain (cervical spine or anterior chest or thoracic spine or low back) must be present. In this definition, shoulder and buttock pain is considered as pain for each involved side. "Low back" pain is considered lower segment pain.

2. Pain in 11 of 18 tender point sites on digital palpation.

> *Definition:* Pain, on digital palpation, must be present in at least 11 of the following 18 sites:

> *Occiput:* Bilateral, at the suboccipital muscle insertions.
> *Low cervical:* bilateral, at the anterior aspects of the intertransverse spaces at C5-C7.
> *Trapezius:* bilateral, at the midpoint of the upper border.
> *Supraspinatus:* bilateral, at origins, above the scapula spine near the medial border.
> *Second rib:* bilateral, at the second costochondral junctions, just lateral to the junctions on upper

surfaces.

Lateral epicondyle: bilateral, 2 cm distal to the epicondyles.

Gluteal: bilateral, in upper outer quadrants of buttocks in anterior fold of muscle.

Greater trochanter: bilateral, posterior to the trochanteric prominence.

Knee: bilateral, at the medial fat pad proximal to the joint line.

Digital palpation should be performed with an approximate force of 4 kg.

For a tender point to be considered "positive" the subject must state that the palpation was painful. "Tender is not to be considered "painful."

http://www.rheumatology.org/publications/classification/fi bromyalgia/fibro.asp

There is *still no gold standard for making a diagnosis of fibromyalgia,* but there is an increasing consensus for the development of new guidelines for diagnosis that modifies the currently proscribed tender point evaluation[6]. *[Italics and bold added by this author.]*

Rough Fibromyalgia Epidemiology

"Fibromyalgia affects 2 to 4 percent of the U.S. population, and it predominantly affects women. "Fibromyalgia affects three times as many women as men," says Dr. Jacob Teitelbaum, medical director of the Fibromyalgia and

Program 120® Team

Fatigue Centers of America and the author of *From Fatigued to Fantastic!* (Avery). Some studies suggest that this number may be closer to ten times as many women as men with the disease, most of who are diagnosed between the ages of 20 and 50[7].

Theories of Causation

Over the years there have been a multitude of theories as to the cause and the definition of fibromyalgia. As the term implies, it was logically thought to be a muscle disease, since muscle pain seemed to be the primary symptom. But the root cause did not seem to lie in the muscles. For a while, it was theorized that it might be an autoimmune disorder, but once again research revealed no root cause disturbance initiating in the immune system.

Sadly for most of the past 200 years, fibromyalgia was thought to be a psychiatric or psychosomatic disorder. This often happens when medical science cannot identify an illness using technology of the day. Even today, there are a lot of medical professionals who insist on hanging on to this theory[8].

For the most part, the symptoms of fibromyalgia can be traced to pituitary dysfunction. Modern medical literature strongly indicates this as the root cause.

In my work, I encounter a large number of patients who relate experiences with other physicians who think their symptoms are mental or psychosomatic. These patients are prescribed psychotropic medications. I also see patients who are put on huge amounts of pain medication (narcotics), seizure medication (not to treat seizures, but to try to deal with neuropathic problems), sleep medications, and so forth. After nearly a year of proper therapy, I have almost no patients who continue on any of these medications.

A big part of the problem with fibromyalgia treatment and diagnosis is a lack of proper communication among various specialties. This is not unlike what happened leading up to and after the 9/11 terror incidents when the various intelligence agencies were not adequately and properly sharing information. There is also a lack of one key specialty that should be the expert in treating fibromyalgia – pituitary endocrinology.

That said, I know that every patient is as different as a snowflake. You cannot put them all into one box and say "Ah hah! This is indeed the exact problem!" Every patient has a different background genetically, slightly different damage to their pituitary and secondary endocrine organs, and different length of time they have had the injury. Instead of a solo musician, this disease is like a symphony – a complex one that sounds different to each patient. The issues that cascade from the injury of this small organ, *the master hormone gland*, can be the writer of this tragic and complex symphony of interactions.

This is what I believe causes fibromyalgia – anterior and/or posterior pituitary dysfunction.

Chapter 3
Etiology of Fibromyalgia

Etiology or Causes According to the Literature

1. Heavy Metal Poisoning
2. Chronic Viral Infection
3. Pituitary Dysfunction/Damage

(Remember, according to medical literature, this is a disorder of "unknown cause.")

Heavy Metal Poisoning

Heavy metals (lead, mercury, etc.) should be a consideration, but only as a tertiary possibility. The literature is thin on this topic, but the excellent work by Dietrich Klinghardt, MD, Ph.D.[9] and others[10] have presented this as a possibility. The laboratory tests ordered for heavy metal poisoning are often incredibly expensive (and perhaps the reason it is considered by less knowledgeable practitioners). Outside of Dr. Klinghardt's work there is only mild support in the literature beyond a few scant articles.

Chelation Therapy

Doctors hear "Can I get the metals cleaned out my arteries through chelation therapy?"

Numerous studies have shown chelation therapies with EDTA have typically NOT worked[11]. They have, on the other hand, been associated with death.

A recently completed trial[12], however, may have shown that EDTA-tetracycline combination can reduce the calcification found in advanced cases. This was not an actual chelation trial, but did use EDTA similar to chelation therapy. (One hundred patients with stable CAD and positive CAC scores were enrolled into a four month study of comET therapy. ComET therapy is composed of (1) Nutraceutical Powder (Vitamin C, Vitamin B6, Niacin, Folic Acid, Selenium, EDTA, l-Arginine, l-Lysine, l-Ornithine, Bromelain, Trypsin, CoQ10, Grapeseed Extract, Hawthorn Berry, Papain) 5cm (3) taken orally every evening; (2) Tetracycline HCl 500mg taken orally every evening; (3) EDTA 1500mg taken in a rectal suppository base every evening).

Treatment, if considered, (or if you just wish to cover your bases), would be with EDTA[13] which binds the heavy metals and will cause patients to pass them through their kidneys. Patients can take it orally or in suppositories.

My research team has recently developed and patented a new topical glutathione that is now seemingly the only true stable reduced glutathione that is easily available to the public. Glutathione is a very sticky molecule (also the body's most potent anti-oxidant) and aggressively binds up for urinary excretion any heavy metals or noxious substances. There are 89,000 articles on PubMed about

GSH (Glutathione) including several NIH review articles worth looking at in detail.

Chronic Viral or Bacterial Infections

The relationship between chronic infection and fibromyalgia is unclear. There are huge numbers of articles with no consensus. Several sources have been studied; Hep C[14], HTLC1[15], Hepatitis B[16], Parvovirus, H1N1, and Lyme disease. These, and others, are all considered to be culprits.

"In addition, there has been interest throughout the past ten years in infectious diseases including hepatitis C, Lyme disease, coxsackie B, HIV, and parvovirus infection, which may cause or trigger fibromyalgia[17]."

These studies all vaguely support (some not as strongly[18]) viral or infectious causation of fibromyalgia, but I'm not convinced. From a pituitary dysfunction perspective (and according to my own clinical experience) infections can "cause" fibromyalgia from the damage they do to the pituitary during hypotensive episodes or shock. Some patients had pituitary dysfunction and *then* secondary immune system suppression opened them up to a higher risk for infection. In this situation the infection comes from pituitary dysfunction, it doesn't cause pituitary dysfunction. The infection is found by happenstance during the work-up of the fibromyalgia.

Real Fibromyalgia Rx – A Pituitary Perspective

Clearly severe viral infections (hemorrhagic fever[19], Puumula Virus[20]) can cause panhypopituitarism, but these viruses are fairly rare in the western world.

Treatment – Viral Valtrex® (valacyclovir)— Valacyclovir is used to slow down genital herpes, but is also often the drug of choice for the treatment of "viral fibromyalgia." I'm not sure why. I believe the reasoning behind its use is anecdotal.

Refer to a study from 2004: **J Rheumatol. 2004 Apr; 31 (4): 783-4.**

No effect of antiviral (valacyclovir) treatment in fibromyalgia: a double blind, randomized study.

Kendall SA, Schaadt ML, Graff LB, Wittrup I, Malmskov H, Krogsgaard K, Bartels EM, Bliddal H, Danneskiold-Samsøe B.

Parker Institute, Department of Rheumatology, Frederiksberg Hospital, Frederiksberg, Denmark.

OBJECTIVE: To investigate the effect of an antiviral compound, valacyclovir, on pain and tenderness in patients with the fibromyalgia (FM) syndrome. METHODS: Sixty patients were randomized into a double blind, placebo controlled 6 week trial. Primary outcome was pain intensity change (on visual analog scale). Secondary outcome measures were tender points (myalgic score) and Fibromyalgia Impact Questionnaire (FIQ). RESULTS: Fifty-two patients completed the study. The numbers of dropouts due to adverse events were equal in valacyclovir (2) and placebo (2) groups. The effect of valacyclovir on pain and tenderness and FIQ did not differ from placebo.

CONCLUSION: Valacyclovir cannot be recommended as a therapy for FM at this point.

Fibromyalgia; a true etiology

Remember the complex symphony of causation of fibromyalgia? I've already said that I believe pituitary dysfunction or damage is the cause of fibromyalgia. This is not a new theory, but one that's been pretty thoroughly researched. The literature is fairly clear about this (once you work through a crazy patchwork of assumptions, presumptions, and theories). I believe that the real problem is a lack of communication among the few pituitary endocrinologists out there. Admittedly these professionals are overworked, few in number, and mostly concerned with other matters.

Here's what is being said in the literature:

In **1998:** "it seems reasonable to suggest that there may be some relationship between basal and dynamic function of the HPA axis and clinical manifestations of FM and CFS[21]."

In **2000:** "Further study of specific components of the HPA axis should ultimately clarify the reproducible

23

abnormalities associated with a clinical picture of CFS. The authors conclude that the observed pattern of hormonal deviations in patients with FMS is a CNS adjustment to chronic pain and stress, constitutes a specific entity of FMS, and is primarily evoked by activated CRH *[Corticotropin-releasing hormone]* neurons.[22]"

In **2007:** "The hypothalamo-pituitary-adrenal (HPA) axis plays a major role in the regulation of responses to stress. Human stress-related disorders such as chronic fatigue syndrome (CFS), fibromyalgia syndrome (FMS), chronic pelvic pain and post-traumatic stress disorder are characterized by alterations in HPA axis activity. However, the role of the HPA axis alterations in these stress-related disorders is not clear. **Most studies have shown that the HPA axis is underactive in the stress-related disorders, but contradictory results have also been reported, which may be due to the patients selected for the study, the methods used for the investigation of the HPA axis, the stage of the syndrome when the tests have been done and the interpretation of the results**[23]"

Clearly there's an issue with knowing whether long-term HPA problems (i.e. pituitary problems) affect or cause fibromyalgia. I believe it lies at the root of most cases of fibromyalgia. There is nothing else in the literature that is consistently supported. I researched this area on PubMed for months. There is nothing else.

Problems lie in the fact that all cases are unique, that all training is a little different, and that there are very few pituitary endocrinologists (let's call them "above-the-neck" endocrinologists).

The study done in 2007 noted that there were problems with the patients selected. Is it possible to change this? Every patient is a snowflake. There were problems with the methods used (labs, values, Tesla ratings of the various MRI's). There were problems with the stage per length of time for the pituitary damage to sit there untreated (sometimes for decades), and again, problems with the interpretation of the results.

Can you see the problem? Half of the conclusions in studies I looked at are backwards. Often it's an issue of which came first, the chicken or the egg?

Why Fibromyalgia Occurs

Anterior pituitary damage causes all kinds of issues downstream in the body – the effects are huge and lifelong.

Below are listed some of these issues from most likely to least likely after any form of TBI (even mild):

Decreased HGH production affects the ability to enter REM and Stage IV sleep[24][25] and to heal muscles[26], nerves[27], and joints[28]. This is a huge problem – lack of effective quality sleep is one of the biggest complaints I hear.

Decreased LH production affects the gonad's (ovaries or testicles) ability to produce testosterone. This is also called central or secondary hypogonadism (primary hypogonadism occurs when the testicles or ovaries themselves are affected). Low testosterone in general causes fatigue[29], a decreased ability of the muscles and tendons to heal[30], weakens the heart, and leads to vascular inflammation[31] and thus CAD (coronary artery disease – the cause of heart attacks and strokes). Specifically, low testosterone in men also causes a decrease in muscles, causes muscle wasting (i.e. sarcopenia[32]), migraine headaches in men[33] (and some women but almost always *the real cause* of migraines in men), and a photophobia (bright lights or sunlight bothers eyes). It also affects nerve myelination. Lack of testosterone can cause a demyelination[34], which can lead to numbness and tingling in the feet, toes and fingers.

Decreased FSH production affects progesterone levels which causes migraines[35], PMS[36], hot flashes and night sweats[37], and affects ovulation. Low FSH in men causes a decrease in sperm and spermatic fluid production[38]. This lack of progesterone in turn (and especially in fibromyalgia) can cause a demyelination[39]. This is critical to many fibromyalgia problems. It can lead to numbness and tingling in the feet, toes, and fingers and can cause gut problems (from a Vagal Nerve demyelination). A lack of progesterone causes migraine headaches in women because of vascular inflammation. The inflammation can also cause strokes and heart attacks (myocardial infarction). Progesterone helps to reduce vascular inflammation[40].

Decreased TSH production affects thyroid production of T4, which leads to fatigue[41], cold extremities[42], brittle fragile hair and hair loss in women[43].

Decreased ACTH production if there's posterior pituitary damage (to the back side of the pituitary) decreases cortisol production from the adrenals. This in turn causes hypocortisolism or even Addison's Disease, hypotension, then fibromyalgia[44], and horrible fatigue.

Chapter 4
Causes and Diagnosis of Adrenal Insufficiency

The cause of secondary adrenal insufficiency

*From **endocrine.niddk.nih.gov**:*

"Secondary adrenal insufficiency can be traced to a lack of ACTH. Without ACTH to stimulate the adrenal glands, the adrenals' production of cortisol drops. Aldosterone production is not usually affected.

A temporary form of secondary adrenal insufficiency may occur when a person who has been taking a synthetic glucocorticoid hormone such as prednisone for a long time stops taking the medication, either abruptly or gradually. Glucocorticoid hormones, which are often used to treat inflammatory illnesses such as rheumatoid arthritis, asthma, and ulcerative colitis, block the release of both CRH (corticotropin-releasing hormone) and ACTH. As a result, the adrenals may begin to atrophy—or shrink—from lack of ACTH stimulation and then fail to secrete sufficient levels of cortisol.

A person who stops taking a synthetic glucocorticoid hormone may have enough ACTH to function when healthy. However, when a person is under the stress of an illness, accident, or surgery, the person's body may not have enough ACTH to stimulate the adrenal glands to produce cortisol.

Another cause of secondary adrenal insufficiency is surgical removal of the noncancerous, ACTH-producing tumors of the pituitary gland that cause Cushing's disease. Cushing's disease is another disorder that leads to excess cortisol in the body. In this case, the source of ACTH is suddenly removed and replacement hormone must be taken until normal ACTH and cortisol production resumes.

Less commonly, adrenal insufficiency occurs when the pituitary gland either decreases in size or stops producing ACTH. These events can result from

- tumors or infections of the area
- loss of blood flow to the pituitary
- radiation for the treatment of pituitary tumors
- surgical removal of parts of the hypothalamus
- surgical removal of the pituitary gland

Diagnosing adrenal insufficiency

In its early stages, adrenal insufficiency can be difficult to diagnose. A review of a patient's medical history and symptoms may lead a doctor to suspect Addison's disease.

A diagnosis of adrenal insufficiency is confirmed through laboratory tests. The aim of these tests is first to determine whether levels of cortisol are insufficient and then to establish the cause. Radiologic exams of the adrenal and pituitary glands also are useful in helping to establish the cause.

Real Fibromyalgia Rx – A Pituitary Perspective

ACTH [Adrenocorticotropic hormone] Stimulation Test

The ACTH stimulation test is the most commonly used test for diagnosing adrenal insufficiency. In this test, blood cortisol, urine cortisol, or both are measured before and after a synthetic form of ACTH is given by injection. The normal response after an ACTH injection is a rise in blood and urine cortisol levels. People with Addison's disease or long-standing secondary adrenal insufficiency have little or no increase in cortisol levels.

Both low- and high-dose ACTH stimulation tests may be used depending on the suspected cause of adrenal insufficiency. For example, if secondary adrenal insufficiency is mild or of recent onset, the adrenal glands may still respond to ACTH because they have not yet atrophied. Some studies suggest a low dose—1 microgram—may be more effective in detecting secondary adrenal insufficiency because the low dose is still enough to raise cortisol levels in healthy people but not in people with mild or recent secondary adrenal insufficiency.

CRH [Corticotropin-releasing hormone] Stimulation Test

When the response to the ACTH test is abnormal, a CRH stimulation test can help determine the cause of adrenal insufficiency. In this test, synthetic CRH is injected intravenously and blood cortisol is measured before and 30, 60, 90, and 120 minutes after the injection. People with Addison's disease respond by producing high levels of ACTH but no cortisol. People with secondary adrenal insufficiency have absent or delayed ACTH responses. CRH will not stimulate ACTH secretion if the pituitary is damaged, so an absent ACTH response points to the pituitary as the cause. A delayed ACTH response points to the hypothalamus as the cause.

Diagnosis During an Emergency

If patients are suspected of having an Addisonian crisis, health professionals must begin treatment with injections of salt, glucose-containing fluids, and glucocorticoid hormones immediately. Although a reliable diagnosis is not possible during crisis treatment, measurement of blood ACTH and cortisol during the crisis—before glucocorticoids are given—is enough to make a preliminary diagnosis. Low blood sodium, low blood glucose, and high blood potassium are also usually present at the time of an adrenal crisis. Once the crisis is controlled, an ACTH stimulation test can be performed to obtain the specific diagnosis. More complex laboratory tests are sometimes used if the diagnosis remains unclear.

Other Tests

Once a diagnosis of Addison's disease is made, radiologic studies such as an x ray or an ultrasound of the abdomen may be taken to see if the adrenals have any signs of calcium deposits. Calcium deposits may indicate bleeding in the adrenal gland or TB, for which a tuberculin skin test also may be used. Blood tests can detect antibodies associated with autoimmune Addison's disease.

If secondary adrenal insufficiency is diagnosed, doctors may use different imaging tools to reveal the size and shape of the pituitary gland. The most common is the computerized tomography (CT) scan, which produces a series of x-ray pictures giving cross-sectional images. A magnetic resonance imaging (MRI) scan may also be used to produce a three-dimensional image of this region. The function of the pituitary and its ability to produce other hormones also are assessed with blood tests.

Treating adrenal insufficiency

Treatment of adrenal insufficiency involves replacing, or substituting, the hormones that the adrenal glands are not making. Cortisol is replaced with a synthetic glucocorticoid such as hydrocortisone, prednisone, or dexamethasone, taken orally one to three times each day, depending on which medication is chosen. If aldosterone is also deficient, it is replaced with oral doses of a mineralocorticoid, called fludrocortisone acetate (Florinef), taken once or twice a day. Doctors usually advise patients receiving aldosterone replacement therapy to increase their salt intake. Because people with secondary adrenal insufficiency normally maintain aldosterone production, they do not require aldosterone replacement therapy. The doses of each medication are adjusted to meet the needs of the individual.

During an Addisonian crisis, low blood pressure, low blood glucose, and high levels of potassium can be life threatening. Standard therapy involves intravenous injections of glucocorticoids and large volumes of intravenous saline solution with dextrose, a type of sugar. This treatment usually brings rapid improvement. When the patient can take fluids and medications by mouth, the amount of glucocorticoids is decreased until a maintenance dose is reached. If aldosterone is deficient, maintenance therapy also includes oral doses of fludrocortisone acetate.

Special problems with adrenal insufficiency

Surgery

Because cortisol is a "stress hormone," people with chronic adrenal insufficiency who need any type of surgery requiring general anesthesia must be treated with intravenous glucocorticoids and saline. Intravenous treatment begins before surgery and continues until the patient is fully awake after surgery and able to take medication by mouth. The "stress" dosage is adjusted as the patient recovers until the presurgery maintenance dose is reached.

In addition, people who are not currently taking glucocorticoids but who have taken long-term glucocorticoids in the past year should tell their doctor before surgery. These people may have sufficient ACTH for normal events, but they may need intravenous treatment for the stress of surgery.

Illness

During illness, oral dosing of glucocorticoid may be adjusted to mimic the normal response of the adrenal glands to this stress on the body. Significant fever or injury may require triple oral dosing. Once recovery from the stress event is achieved, dosing is then returned to maintenance levels. People with adrenal insufficiency should know how to increase medication during such periods of stress. Immediate medical attention is needed if severe infections, vomiting, or diarrhea occur. These conditions can precipitate an Addisonian crisis.

Pregnancy

Women with adrenal insufficiency who become pregnant are treated with standard replacement therapy. If nausea and vomiting in early pregnancy interfere with taking medication by mouth, injections of the hormone may be necessary. During delivery, treatment is similar to that of people needing surgery. Following delivery, the dose is gradually tapered until the usual maintenance doses of oral hydrocortisone are reached.

How can someone with adrenal insufficiency prepare for an emergency?

People with adrenal insufficiency should always carry identification stating their condition in case of an emergency. A card or medical alert tag should notify emergency health care providers of the need to inject cortisol if the person is found severely injured or unable to answer questions. The card or tag should also include the name and telephone number of the person's doctor and the name and telephone number of a family member to be notified. The dose of hydrocortisone needed may vary with a person's age or size. For example, a child younger than 2 years of age can receive 25 milligrams (mg), a child between 2 and 8 years of age can receive 50 mg, and a child older than 8 years should receive the adult dose of 100 mg. When traveling, people with adrenal insufficiency should carry a needle, syringe, and an injectable form of cortisol for emergencies."

http://endocrine.niddk.nih.gov/pubs/addison/addison.htm. Accessed March 11, 2010.

Chapter 5
How Fibromyalgia Occurs; pituitary damage causes a cascade of hormone problems

The pituitary is fragile – one of the most critical organs in the body is located at one of the weakest points of the body. It is the master hormone gland and controls almost everything, either directly or indirectly.

Below is a list of problems that can cause stalk or pituitary damage. Look for these in your history:

- Whiplash[45] or any motor vehicle accident
- TBI – even mild[46]
- Air bag deployment to face or head
- Any mild or moderate blow to the head – heading a soccer ball, any concussion.[47]
- Sexual abuse as a child[48]
- Stroke[49]
- Tumors[50] – if you can't find anything else[51].
- Sheehan's Syndrome[52] – most common in Utah
- Snorting or huffing drugs (i.e. cocaine, meth)[53]
- Radiation exposure[54] (common in medical professions)
- Prolonged High Stress[55] (common in medical professions)

The Anatomy of the Pituitary – it's very fragile.

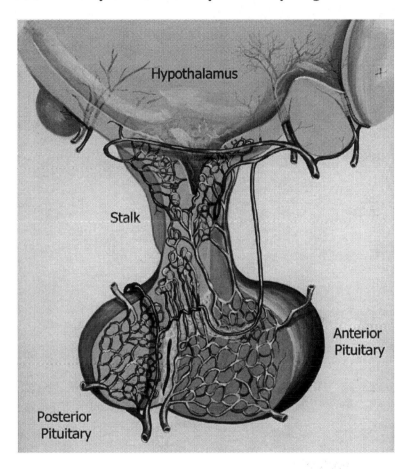

Pituitary Picture – note all the fragile vasculature. *(Painted in oil by illustrator Janel Jensen of Provo, Utah.)*

Real Fibromyalgia Rx – A Pituitary Perspective

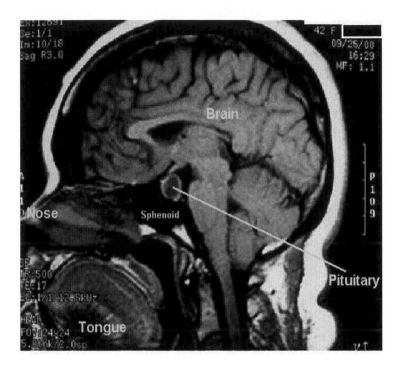

MRI of the pituitary

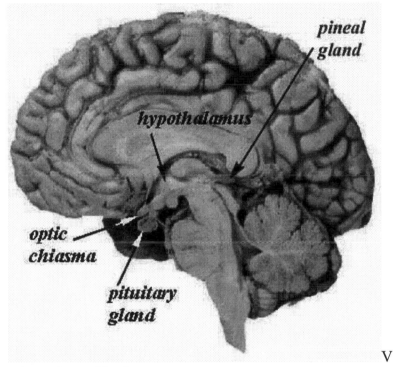

View of a real brain.

Why is Fibromyalgia Seven Times More Common Among Women?

Why are more women diagnosed with fibromyalgia than men? Simple – men die before they get in to see a doctor. For men with fibromyalgia, low testosterone and/or HGH and hypothyroidism cause a sludgy hyperlipemic blood, which leads to a much higher risk of CAD (which causes heart attacks) and/or strokes[56]. Men are at higher risk of these anyway. Women with fibromyalgia live and suffer on. The little bit of progesterone and estradiol female fibromyalgia patients make seems to protect them from strokes and heart attacks[57], so they live longer.

The Double Whammy Patient and What It Means

"Double Whammy" patients describes women who have been suffering from mild to moderate fibromyalgia for years, but as they reach menopause (average age of 51 for white females in America), their symptoms get worse. This decline happens because of the menopause-induced loss of progesterone, estradiol, and testosterone. The healing benefits they derive[58] from those hormones are lost. A mild case of fibromyalgia suddenly becomes a severe and debilitating case.

This confirms that fibromyalgia is mostly hormonal in etiology and that the premise for this book is indeed correct and accurate.

Estradiol

Women make 17β-estradiol in their ovaries. Estrogens and 17β-estradiol are very healing[59] [60] and beneficial for women. From 17β-estradiol comes all the necessary downstream estrogens women need (except estrone which is created in the gut).

From my *Program 120® Handbook* for physicians:

Program 120® Team

Estrogen (Usually Estradiol and Estriol)

(Note: Only for surgical or FSH-elevated (>50 mIU/ml[61]) confirmed menopause.)

Human estrogen is produced in four different forms[62] – estrone (E1), estradiol (E2), estriol (E3), and estetrol (E4 -- in pregnancy only). Estradiol is the most physiologically and biologically active and the one which offers the most protection and benefits – it also converts to estrone which, along with estradiol, also converts to estriol. So technically and theoretically (if the patient is young enough to have all their CYP3A7 cytochrome P-450 16-hydroxylation liver conversion enzymes remaining intact[63]) it can be the only estrogen you need to give. But usually this form of HRT is given orally or transdermally (only in certain situations) as a bi-estrogen, or BiEst, containing both estradiol and estriol, or more specifically, human 17β-estradiol which can also be given in a compounded form or as Estrace® at 1 mgm a day which usually gives high enough levels to give proper cardiovascular protection[64]. Many people believe that estriol protects against cancer but there have been no studies to prove this.

Dosing and Manner

Most often it should be given orally in a capsule (safer for the heart and breasts but slightly higher risk of gallstones[65]) as compounded Bi-Est in the morning consisting of a beginning dose of 0.5 mgm of estriol and 1.0 mgm of estradiol. We also know now that you can give your

41

patients pure compounded 17β-estradiol (E2) at either 1.0-2.0 mgm or as Estrace® 1.0 mgm a day. The estradiol level can be raised to 1.5 mgm, or 2.0 mgm or decreased to 0.5 mgm but always keep it (you can choose not to give the estriol for a number of good reasons).

Note that estriol (E3) is the breakdown product of estradiol (E2) and because of this does not actually have to be given.

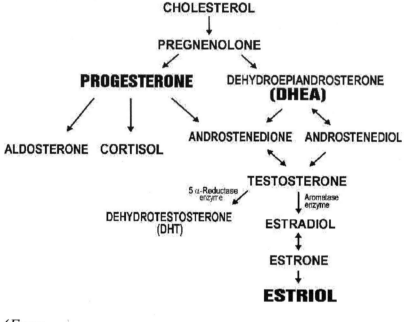

(From http://lib.store.yahoo.net/lib/gentlepharmacy/hormone-biopath.jpg)

Oral Estrogen CVD Warnings

ORAL ESTROGEN WARNING #1 -- Prothrombin 20210G→A Variant Warning

Do not EVER give oral estradiol to women who are *postmenopausal with essential hypertension* because a high percentage of these particular hypertensive women will have a prothrombin clotting factor genetic variant[66] (mutation) and could suffer from VTE/DVT, MI (332 percent increased risk[67]), or stroke[68]. Though oral is clearly the best option, with these particular patients instead give them a transdermal estradiol patch[69] (to protect their skin and mucosa and some bone protection only, but at least transdermal will protect that[70]).

(For the technically minded this is the Prothrombin 20210G→A Variant[71].)

Do not give or allow to be given oral estrogen to these women (if these are your patients, stop the oral estrogen and switch them to transdermal BiEst or the Climara® patch).

ORAL ESTROGEN WARNING #2 – The Oral Estradiol Window!

We do know from HERS, the Nurses' Health Study, and the WHI that there is a **window of opportunity for safely starting oral estradiol[72]** in postmenopausal women starting within a year after they become menopausal (average age in the United States is 51) and going up to age

60, after which they are at increased risk for the first year of oral estradiol for a myocardial infarction[73]. Use extreme caution and have them sign an informed consent/release if they still want oral estradiol and are willing to face the risks involved. Otherwise use topical, transdermal Bi-Est or transdermal Estrace® or an estradiol ring in these women *(see below)*.

We know however those endogenous AND exogenous estrogens, such as estradiol, protect the cardiovascular system, and several observational studies and a few small clinical studies conducted *in healthy and younger postmenopausal women* (i.e. under 60) support this hypothesis[74].

However if these older women are already more than a year on oral estrogens or have a long history of being on estrogen, it is far more beneficial and cardioprotective, neuroprotective, and osteoprotective for them to continue the oral estrogens.

Article In Support of Oral Estrogen Warnings

Read the following landmark articles if you disagree with these warnings.

Differential association of oral and transdermal oestrogen-replacement therapy with venous thromboembolism risk by Pierre-Yves Scarabin, et al in The Lancet 2003; 362:428-432.

Hormone Replacement Therapy, Prothrombotic Mutations, and the Risk of Incident Nonfatal Myocardial Infarction in Postmenopausal Women by Bruce M. Psaty, MD, PhD et al. in JAMA. 2001;285:906-913.

Alternatives to Oral Estrogen Therapy by Valerie L. Baker, MD in Obstetrics and Gynecology Clinics of North America, Vol. 21, No. 2, June 1994, pp. 271-97.

Levels

For a NEWLY menopausal woman you want treated estradiol levels to be 75-100 pg/mL or slightly greater.

For an OLDER menopausal woman you want treated estradiol levels to be >50 pg/mL or slightly greater (JT Hargrove et al suggested levels of 50-150 pg/ml[75] but we'd keep it below 100 pg/ml to prevent estrogen predominance symptoms).

Levels should be maintained above 50 pg/ml (to 100 pg/ml) to keep patients feeling the best physically[76] and psychologically[77].

In humans, the epidemiological studies have shown that premenopausal women have a much lower mortality from atherosclerotic cardiovascular disease than men, suggesting that sex hormones might have a cardioprotective effect[78].

Real Fibromyalgia Rx – A Pituitary Perspective

Simple Point on Biologically Identical Human Estrogens

Bio-identical Human Estrogens (not patentable because we all manufacture in our body)

vs.

Synthetic Estrogens (patentable)

Any questions?

Effects of No Estrogen

1. Vaginal dryness and atrophy[79]
2. Urinary incontinence[80]
3. Hot flashes[81] that do not resolve with progesterone (use supraphysiological doses)
4. Temperature dysregulation
5. Balance problems
6. Sagging wrinkled skin[82]
7. Sagging breasts[83]
8. Epidermal thinning, declining dermal collagen content, diminished skin moisture, decreased laxity, and impaired wound healing[84]
9. Fatigue[85]
10. Depression[86]
11. Mood swings[87]
12. Declining libido to no libido
13. Acceleration of glomerulosclerosis
14. Osteoporosis[88]

15. Coronary artery disease[89]
16. Sexual dysfunction[90]
17. Tooth loss and receding gums [91].
18. Alzheimer's Disease[92]

Benefits Of Human Bi-Estrogen (ERT: Estradiol and Estriol: E2 and E3) or Estradiol (E2 or Estrace®)

1. Estrogen supplementation prevents macular degeneration[93].
2. Estrogen supplementation prevents cataracts[94].
3. Estrogen supplementation prevents memory loss and Alzheimer's disease[95].
4. Estrogen prevents osteoporosis[96].
5. Estrogen prevents against vaginal atrophy, dry eyes, and skin wrinkling and increases skin thickness in the process[97].
6. Estradiol is cardioprotective by decreasing LDL levels and elevating HDL levels[98][99].
7. Estradiol protects against Ischemic Stroke (contrary to the WHI[100]) (by preventing activation of neutrophils by TNF alpha, thus decreasing the expression of adhesion molecules, the adhesion of neutrophils - endothelial cells, and hence the risk of ischemic stroke)[101].
8. Evidence clearly establishes that estradiol is a potent neuroprotective and neurotrophic factor in the adult: it influences memory and cognition, decreases the risk and delays the onset of neurological diseases such as Alzheimer's disease,

and attenuates the extent of cell death that results from brain injuries such as cerebrovascular stroke and neurotrauma[102].

Direct Antiatherosclerotic Effects[103]

1. Inhibits deposition of LDL and its byproducts in blood vessel walls
2. Decreases lipoprotein-induced arterial smooth muscle proliferation
3. Decreases foam cell formation in vessel wall
4. Reduces arterial cholesterol ester influx and hydrolysis
5. Decreases elastin and collagen production and accumulation
6. Inhibits platelet aggregation
7. Increases prostacyclin production by endothelium and arterial smooth muscle cells
8. Decreases thromboxane A2 formation
9. Reduces oxidation of LDL
10. Protects against vascular injury
11. Accelerates endothelial cell growth and inhibits apoptosis
12. Inhibits proliferation of smooth muscle cells
13. Estrogen-related genes ameliorate negative effects of collagen, E-selectin, vascular endothelial growth factor, and fibrinogen proteins

Program 120® Team

Direct Vasodilatory Effects[104]

1. Decreases vascular tone
2. Modulates release of vasoconstrictors and vasodilators by vascular endothelium, thereby decreasing vascular reactivity
3. Modulates ionic channels in smooth muscle cell membranes of vessels and cardiac cells
4. Modulates release of vasoactive substances and neurotransmitters
5. Modulates vasoactive neurotransmitter release at presynaptic junctions
6. Increases vasodilating and antiplatelet aggregation factors in endothelium
7. Increases vasodilatation by nonendothelium-dependent factor
8. Estrogen-related genes ameliorate negative effects of endothelin, prostacyclin synthase, and endothelial nitric oxide

Systemic Effects[105]

1. Decreases total cholesterol and LDL levels; increases HDL levels
2. Increases inotropic actions of the heart
3. Improves glucose metabolism; decreases circulating insulin levels
4. Lowers blood pressure through vasodilatation
5. Reduces plasminogen-activator inhibitor
6. Decreases fibrinogen

Side Effects of Estrogen Dominance or Unopposed Estrogen

1. In Peri-Menopausal patients* with estrogen dominance[106]:
   A. Premenopausal mood swings, depression
   B. Breast swelling, fibrocystic disease
   C. Craving sweets
   D. Heavy or irregular menses
   E. Sleep disturbances: Insomnia or fatigue
   F. Uterine fibroids
   G. Weight gain, fat deposition on hips and thighs
   H. Acne and skin breaks out
   I. Water retention, edema

*This can continue for years, starting in a patient's late 30s to menopause in their early 50s. Realize that the estrogen dominance effect can be overwhelming and long lasting. It has an overwhelming effect on their risk factors for breast and endometrial cancer. Offset it with adequate human progesterone.

2. **The Five B's of Estrogen Dominance** (can occur with PMS* [Pre-Menstrual Syndrome] or with PMS* [Peri-Menopausal Symptoms]):
   A. Backache
   B. Bleeding (excessively)
   C. Bloating
   D. Breast (tenderness)
   E. Bitchiness

At the request of the gynecologists on the Program 120® Team I'll add a tentative sixth item – Uterine Fibroids.)

*Treat Pre-Menstrual Syndrome and Peri-Menopausal Symptoms the same way. Both are caused by estrogen dominance or over-production (which can also predispose them to breast cancer and endometrial hyperplasia. *Physicians, ask if their mom had this and did she have breast CA or uterine cancer.* Give them 100 mgm progesterone triturates for sublingual dissolution for whenever they start to have these symptoms. If it doesn't work, try two each day. If two doesn't work, try three! If three doesn't work, try four! (*Oral* human progesterone or P4 is a sedative and soporific, while this is not true of the sublingual triturates.)

3. Breast Cancer[107]
4. Endometrial Cancer[108]
5. Thrombosis[109]
6. Weight gain[110] – debatable (exercise helps – do lots of it!)
7. Fluid retention[111] – use Dyazide
8. Uterine Fibroids (Uterine Leiomyomas)[112]
9. Migraine Headache[113]
10. Gallstones – when given orally[114]
11. Heart Attack (HERS study[115] – wrong kinds of estrogen though [i.e. CEE])
12. Tooth loss and jaw resorption[116]
13. Depressed mood[117]

Real Fibromyalgia Rx – A Pituitary Perspective

How to Fix Side Effects of Estrogen Dominance

If the patient is premenopausal or perimenopausal or even premenstrual syndrome (all the types of PMS out there), give them 100 mgm progesterone triturates (see Progesterone info below) for sublingual dissolution for whenever they start to have these symptoms.

If you see these symptoms in someone who's post-menopausal and on modern HRT, lower the dose of estradiol in the BiEst you are giving. If that doesn't work, keep the dose low, but cut out the Estriol (E3) portion.

Practice Gems on Estrogen Supplementation

1. Protect your patient from cancers, cataracts and heart disease – it is your obligation – give them proper HRT protection.

2. Take E2 and E3 as a micronized capsule. Give them Estrace® 1 mg a day if their insurance will cover it. Give them generic Estrace® if finances are an issue.

3. Ask your patients if they want to be dried up like a prune and have incredibly wrinkled skin, no teeth, and no sex – or would they like some estrogen?

4. **Pre-/Perimenopausal Situations**: look at FSH levels which go up and down. If premenopausal, you can give progesterone only (one tablet a day). They make plenty of estrogen naturally. No use checking levels of estradiol or progesterone in these patients. If

perimenopausal, check FSH levels. If high then treat, if not high (low) you can use progesterone – no harm in giving progesterone to an anovulatory perimenopausal woman. If they want to bleed (ask them), just stop the progesterone – if they don't want to bleed, continue the progesterone. After 3 to 6 months stop the progesterone, after one month check a FSH level to see where they are.

5. It does no good to measure pre-menopausal estradiol and progesterone levels because you don't know where they are in their cycle. Check FSH and LH levels instead, if you are concerned.

6. You can diagnose menopause by symptoms – if no menses for six (6) months it's menopause. This goes for almost any age, any symptoms. If they request it, you'd better suspect it. Measure the FSH and LH (menopause if both are >50).

7. Use human biologically identical hormones, not equine urine estrones which (as we've said repeatedly) contain 17 androgenic and carcinogenic agents.

8. I tried a tri-estrogen combination first, but it had too many side effects (our female patients make enough estrone anyway). I use a BiEst (bi-estrogen or two estrogens) containing both estradiol (20 percent) and estriol (80 percent) in doses such as 1.5 mgm, 2.0 mgm, or 2.5 mgm (usually contains only 0.5 mgm estriol). Even easier, just use estradiol (such as Estrace® 1 mg).

9. Do not use estrone. Not breast tissue friendly. This is already created in the stomach lining to such an extent that most women are never short of estrone.

10. If you have a patient on HRT, you should aggressively communicate the need for PAP and breast mammograms – every two years according to the American Cancer Association and ACOG (if they are past age 40) but annually if in on HRT. Send out letters. Do whatever is necessary.

MALPRACTICE WARNING: Do not refill HRT unless they comply!

11. Don't guess. Check levels! **Optimal estradiol level is 50-100 pg/ml**. You can get annoying side effects if above 100 (breast tenderness, vaginal bleeding, bloating, breaking out), but must be at least 50 pg/ml to give protection.

12. No need to cycle estradiol after menopause – give every day!

13. If they have had their uterus or ovaries removed then give them everything – BiEst, Testosterone, DHEA, and Progesterone. Save their lives!

14. MALPRACTICE WARNING: Absolute contraindications – history of clots, thrombosis, emboli, or HTN (hypertension). DO NOT GIVE THESE PATIENTS ORAL ESTROGEN! Give them an estradiol patch (Climara®) (and Niaspan® 500 mgm

BID) or an estrogen ring (see below). Note that patch does not help as strongly against CV disease[118] as oral.

15. If they have hot flashes that are not resolved, go to BID with the Bi-Est or Estrace® for six months or so until the symptoms resolve.

16. If they do not have hot flashes until after you start the Bi-Est (or estradiol), then double the dose for six months or so. If this does not resolve the hot flashes, then switch them to a topical patch such as Climara® or Yasmin® (the least androgenic BCPs on the market and for that reason, as this book is written, the *Program 120®* favorite) as BCP can also decrease hot flashes, so try if you're desperate. Know though, that hot flashes are usually caused by perimenopausal decline of the hormone *inhibin*[119].

The other opinion in regards to hot flashes is that in some women catecholestrogens (estrogen metabolites) from oral estrogen[120] "resetting the thermostat" is to blame for hot flashes[121] – if you suspect this is the case, switch them to the Climara® patch for great 24-hour coverage – it's worth a try.

17. Be aware that (very rarely) they can start ovulating on the natural hormones and can get pregnant – warn them if they are younger postmenopausal patients!

18. If the patient is past the window for HRT (age 50-60 years) or has hypertension (thus a prothrombotic risk)

use a vaginal estradiol ring or tablet. Femring® and Vagifem® tablets give proper estradiol levels similar to the Climara® patch while Estring® is for those women with breast cancer, DVT, or MI histories who are having localized vaginal issues (urinary frequency, dry vagina, incontinence, etc.) and in who you do not want circulating estrogens. The Femring®/Vagifem® option can treat hot flashes in some patients (in the occasional instances when progesterone does not).

19. ***Warning***: Estriol (E3) tends to cause bloating or the feeling of bloating. If this occurs among your HRT patients, stop their estriol first. Give a diuretic next (i.e. Dyazide®).

20. There is absolutely no need to check estradiol levels in men. What is being said on the internet is WRONG! If true, at what level would they like the estradiol level to rise before intervention with anastrozole is begun? *[This is a Socratic question – Program 120®]* There is no answer to this, because Estradiol is cardioprotective and prevents against strokes in men[122]. Leave it alone unless they get significant breast enlargement!

Progesterone – Human P4 Benefits

Progesterone (4-pregnene-3, 20-dione or P4 in this case[123]) is the "feel good" hormone of pregnancy. I am talking about naturally occurring biologically identical human progesterone – not synthetic progestational agents such as progestin, medroxyprogesterone acetate, or norethisterone

– these are not the natural progesterone and are problematic. Their side effects are intensive. They have the opposite side effects when compared to the benefits of natural progesterone.

Known Negative Side Effects from Taking Medroxyprogesterone Acetate (MPA)

(Studies are legion, look at Pub Med for more supporting articles) This is by far what most women are given (shockingly) so we'll start here.

MPA is a teratogen and cannot be used in pregnancy[124].

MPA increases cholesterol and increases risk of heart disease[125].

MPA increases foam cell formation, endothelial inflammation, plaque formation, strokes and heart attacks[126].

MPA is carcinogenic and causes breast cancer[127] (see PEPI[128] trial).

MPA has no effect on osteoporosis (i.e. does not help)[129].

MPA is associated with side effects of increased bleeding, bloating, and depression[130].

MPA provides a serum progesterone level of zero – it is immeasurable as progesterone.

MPA *is not progesterone*[131]! *Do not take it (especially if you have fibromyalgia)!*

Known Benefits of Biologically Identical Human Progesterone (P4)

P4, when levels are optimized, aggressively and effectively:

1. Lowers cholesterol *[at 200 mgm of micronized progesterone a day in one PEPI study arm[132] – sound familiar? Program 120®]* Especially when given in conjunction with E2[133].

2. Elevates HDL levels (hard to do)[134].

3. Decreases foam cell formation[135], endothelial inflammation, plaque formation, and thus strokes and heart attacks[136].

4. Decreases breast density and thus breast cancer[137].

5. Increases bone density preventing osteoporosis and related fractures[138].

6. Prevents and treats endometrial hyperplasia (use triple or quadruple the usual dose)[139].

7. If you give enough, progesterone almost always halts uterine bleeding (cyclical bleeding)[140].

8. Can act as a hypersomniac (sleep aid) if you give 100 mgm at night orally for sleep[141] problems. Orally administered progesterone may have advantages over other routes of administration in the treatment of premenstrual syndrome (PMS) because of substantially higher levels of the anxiolytic metabolites 5 alpha and 5 beta pregnenolone[142] which also cause drowsiness[143].

9. Oral P4 also treats peri-menopausal symptoms (also called PMS) in the same manner (give double or triple the usual dose for about a week)[144].

10. Oral micronized progesterone given sublingually has improved bioavailability and fewer reported side effects compared with synthetic progestins[145].

11. P4, when given with estradiol, improves the quality of life according to a Mayo Clinic report[146]

12. Improves libido (along with testosterone)[147].

13. Synthetic progestins, on the other hand, often cause androgenic side effects (acne, body and facial hair), depression, and weight gain. Micronized progesterone is devoid of the androgenic effects on the lipid profile seen with MPA and other synthetic progestational agents; for that reason, it may be preferable in HRT protocols for perimenopausal and postmenopausal women[148].

14. Lack can cause TMJ[149].

15. Demyelination[150] of peripheral nerves or the Vagus or Vagal Nerve (the Tenth or Xth of the twelve cranial nerves but this supplies the heart, the esophagus, stomach, gut and bladder).

16. Men should not take progesterone unless they are a sex offender in jail[151] (see below).

Testosterone Benefits (Male and Female)

Optimized testosterone levels can give your patients:

1. Normal physiological levels increases muscle mass[152]. In my experience it also helps heal muscles.

2. Decreases endothelial resistance acting as a potent vasodilator[153].

3. Higher total testosterone and SHBG (sex hormone binding globulin) levels are inversely related to carotid atherosclerosis, suggesting their potential importance in reducing atherosclerotic risk in postmenopausal women not using HRT[154].

4. Higher free testosterone levels in men are associated with higher cardiac [left ventricle] ejection fractions (higher cardiac output)[155].

5. Age, HDL, and **free testosterone** may be stronger predictors of degree of coronary artery disease than

are blood pressure, cholesterol, diabetes, smoking, and body mass index (BMI)[156].

6. Despite the literature replete with supporting studies[157] [158], cardiologists continue to ignore the favorable benefits of natural testosterone replacement. Don't do the same.

7. There is evidence to suggest that low concentrations of testosterone are associated with an increased risk of CVD in men[159].

8. Testosterone concentration is inversely correlated with procoagulable factors, plasminogen activator inhibitor, and fibrinogen[160]. Give enough testosterone to obtain a good physiologic level and these coagulation factors decline.

9. Testosterone, at physiologic concentrations, induces coronary artery dilation and increases coronary blood flow in men with established coronary artery disease[161].

10. Normal physiological levels improve insulin resistance by bolstering the functionality of insulin receptors[162]. There is an association in men between low concentrations of free and total testosterone and hyperinsulinemia[163].

11. Lower levels predispose to increased BMI and diabetes[164].

12. Normal physiological levels prevent Alzheimer's disease. Low levels of testosterone are an independent risk factor[165]!

13. Normal physiological levels prevent osteoporosis in men and women by increasing bone mineral density (BMD)[166].

14. Normal physiological levels improve erectile dysfunction in men[167].

15. Normal physiological levels improves libido and well-being in men and women (in women who have undergone oophorectomy and hysterectomy, transdermal testosterone improves sexual function and psychological well-being[168].) *As reported in the New England Journal of Medicine using optimized levels from younger women who were menstruating, confirming once again my repeated observation that the peer reviewed studies use the optimized levels and so should the practitioners.*

16. In adult males, testosterone maintains muscle mass and strength, fat distribution, bone mass, erythropoiesis, male hair pattern, libido and potency, and spermatogenesis[169].

17. Testosterone increases HGH production in the elderly – it is critical to create that rich hormonal milieu or stew that allows all eight cylinders of your patient's hormone engines to fire properly. In light

of a Mayo Clinic study showing that giving hypogonadal men, especially elderly men, testosterone causes them to also increase production of endogenous HGH[170]. This is awesome and a heck of a lot cheaper than giving rHGH!

18. 35% of heart patients treated with testosterone *improved* by at least one NYHA (New York Heart Association) class[171].

19. Testosterone replacement therapy improves functional capacity and symptoms in men with moderately severe heart failure[172]. *[Why don't cardiologists put all of their patients on this? – Program 120®]*

20. Testosterone can dramatically improve endurance especially in the frail elderly[173] (but really since it will build muscle and bone mass this can occur at almost any level from age 40 years on[174]).

21. Sex hormones play a key role in numerous physiologic processes and functions and clearly impact wound healing in the all ages of patients[175] but especially the elderly[176].

22. Maintaining appropriate levels until death allows improved cognition, better affect, more rapid thinking/processing skills[177] and decision making and better muscle mass[178].

23. With your erectile dysfunction patients, don't ever give Viagra® until you have worked them up for hypogonadism or testosterone deficiency[179]. Experience shows you will often need to give both testosterone[180] and sildenafil (or your favorite phosphodiesterase inhibitor) to more adequately treat some ED cases.

24. Testosterone in patients can not only improve insulin resistance but increase the number and health of insulin receptors[181]. First, the lack of testosterone in men has been strongly associated with metabolic syndrome[182]. Second, giving testosterone to these men can help clear up the insulin resistance and absolve the pre-diabetic stage[183].

25. Testosterone improves vascular resistance, reduces systolic blood pressure[184], improves dyslipidemias[185] (lowers triglycerides, raises HDL), and improves cardiac output.

26. Normal physiological levels causes improvement in osteoporosis[186] as is clear in a number of studies[187].

27. Testosterone in hypogonadal men improves Alzheimer's disease, Multiple Sclerosis (MS)[188], Huntington's disease[189], Parkinson's disease, and others. As a matter of fact, testosterone loss may be a risk factor for cognitive decline and possibly for dementia[190] and is clearly neuroprotective[191] and

exogenous supplementation proved beneficial for cognitive and brain function in elderly men.

28. Testosterone supplementation can increase red blood cells, an extremely beneficial factor for most older men *and women*, causing a relative erythrocytosis. Do not be mistaken – this is not a polycythemia or a polycythemia vera (see below) – this is just a beneficial erythrocytosis that deserves no treatment, and even minimal observation[192]. Most men *and women* who are hypogonadal are also anemic[193] and supplementing them with testosterone can often resolve this.

29. Testosterone replacement therapy (TRT) improves lower urinary tract symptoms in men (LUTS – urinary frequency, urgency, halting or residual urine in the bladder, etc.) and shrinks benign prostatic hypertrophy (BPH). Erectile dysfunction (ED), which is absolutely associated with hypogonadism or low levels of testosterone, has now been associated with LUTS[194] and BPH[195].

30. In women, testosterone is the main hormone that prevents urogenital and vaginal atrophy – save your female patients from decades of dry vaginas, dry eyes, dry mouth, poor sex lives and embarrassing stress incontinence by giving them a little testosterone just like their ovaries did!

31. Testosterone decline with aging in men is associated with osteoarthritis development[196] and worsening rheumatoid arthritis[197]. Same in women.

32. Testosterone Replacement Therapy (TRT), unlike what is commonly believed is NOT associated with causing frank PIN (prostate intraepithelial neoplasia) to become full prostate cancer. After one year of TRT men with PIN treated at Beth Israel Deaconess Medical Center at the Harvard Medical School do NOT have a greater increase in PSA or a significantly increased risk of cancer than men without PIN. These results indicate that TRT is not contraindicated in men with a history of PIN[198].

33. Contrary to what your local cardiologist says (and some papers erroneously claim as a side effect) physiological testosterone replacement did not adversely affect blood coagulation status (plasminogen activator inhibitor-1 (PAI-1), fibrinogen, tissue plasminogen activator (tPA) and full blood count)[199].

34. Low levels of testosterone in elderly men increase fall risk by 40 percent[200] (probably secondary to weaker antigravity and balance muscles). Fall risk was higher in men with lower bioavailable testosterone levels. The effect of testosterone level was independent of poorer physical performance, suggesting that the effect of testosterone on fall risk may be mediated by other androgen actions.

Cortisol

Lack of cortisol[201] causes fibromyalgia symptoms in some women – hypotension[202], muscle weakness[203], and fatigue. Cortisol comes from the adrenals which are controlled by a tiny area on the rear or back of the pituitary gland and so damage to this area on the pituitary causes lack of these hormones (posterior pituitary dysfunction). But don't get too sidetracked by this hypocortisolism because, in my experience, damaging the back (or rear) of the pituitary is more rare then damaging the front, though I have seen cases where treating isolated hypocortisolism alleviated all of the symptoms of fibromyalgia.

Men (and Some Women) with Fibromyalgia Caused by Pituitary Dysfunction Die from Vascular Disease Early – CAD, Stroke

I see far fewer men than women with fibromyalgia – but I believe they just never get a chance to get it diagnosed – the men with pituitary dysfunction appear to die from coronary artery disease[204] (CAD) and stroke at a much greater frequency then women. The men are dead! This is why there are eight women with fibromyalgia for every man who has it. Lack of these pituitary hormones kills men more quickly while women live on due to protection from their female hormones (estradiol and progesterone).

Chapter 6
Fibromyalgia Signs and Symptoms

Fibromyalgia has a wide array of signs and symptoms that can seem confusing and disparate. I believe they're all related to a cascade of problems that occur – all caused by the same event and root problem – pituitary damage and dysfunction.

Trigger Points

Light microscopic examination revealed no evidence of inflammation. Histochemical analysis demonstrated type II fiber atrophy in seven patients and the "moth-eaten" appearance of type I fibers in five patients. Electron microscopic findings were most impressive, and included **myofibrillar lysis** —

MYOFIBRILLAR = muscle fiber   +   LYSIS = torn

Why does muscle fiber stay torn, and not heal?

Trigger Points: what they are, how they happen and what to do about them

Picture a rubber band with a small section that has lost its elasticity. That section has instead has become hardened and brittle. That's what a trigger point is like. The muscle is tighter, stiffer, and will often be weak and yet tense at the same time. A trigger point (TP) will be sore when you push on it, and you may feel a thick band that you can flick over with your fingers.

A vast number of sports injuries have their genesis in the development of a TP in the muscle or fascia. This is very commonly the first sign of overload. From that point on, cause and effect begin to domino. One tissue breaks down, causing another to be overloaded and break down, and so on. Trigger points lead to inflammation, then pain, then weakness, then joint and nerve dysfunction, and finally structural breakdown of tissues that can keep you out of action for weeks, months or even years. Your recovery will depend on how long you attempt to struggle on without treating the original TP.

A TP is an alarm bell – a first warning sign that things are not well within your biomechanical system. Learning to listen to your body's alarm bells is a critical skill that can help you avoid injuries. Often athletes, with their enhanced overall body sense, become aware of TPs before they are significant enough to cause actual pain (32), when the only complaint is "tightness" or the joint or muscle doesn't "feel right" (20).

http://www.pponline.co.uk/encyc/0703.htm

The definition of TP is widely known in sports injuries, but when it comes to fibromyalgia it seems to be forgotten.

Real Fibromyalgia Rx – A Pituitary Perspective

Treatment

Trigger point injections do not work and are not advisable. A lot of well-meaning physicians have given patients trigger point injections, but in my opinion they are probably not necessary.

Fatigue or Chronic Fatigue Syndrome (CFS)

Why is fatigue associated with fibromyalgia? Hypothyroidism, low testosterone levels (hypogonadism), low cortisol (hypocortisolism), and/or low somatropin (AGHD) are all caused by pituitary dysfunction and can cause fatigue[205].

Most physicians and most labs do not know proper levels and ranges (usually A.A.C.E.). This is problematic. Patients with inappropriate levels aren't treated because their doctor thinks their ranges are normal. This is a tragedy that I see all the time.

The real problem lies in the way most local labs set their ranges (usually skewed low). They usually get a range by taking the last thousand people of a particular sex and age who've been tested, and throw out the top 100 as too high, and the bottom 100 as too low. They determine that the middle 800 have a normal range. This tactic leads them to believe that lower levels are "normal." Their baseline is highly skewed to the low end of the range. What kind of 28-year-old male asks for his testosterone levels to be checked? These men usually have low ranges to begin with, or are being treated and still have low ranges. This is not the proper way to set normative ranges.

Cold Extremities– Almost Never Raynaud's!

Why do some patients have cold extremities (hands and feet)? This may be low tes (hypogonadism[206]) but is usually undiagnosed hypothyroidism[207].

Many people with cold extremities have been diagnosed with Raynaud's. Raynaud's is so rare[208], I've seen very few real cases. I've seen hundreds of patients who have been told they have Raynaud's – especially here in Utah where we have long, cold winters. Truthfully, I don't believe any of these patients actually have Raynaud's, but instead have centrally mediated (pituitary or secondary) hypothyroidism. Treatment is getting their thyroid levels to where they should be.

Hypothyroidism Usually With Thyroid Resistance

Some patients require supraphysiologic doses of thyroid just to feel normal. They report that the thyroid isn't working and they want or need more medication. They have *thyroid resistance* (either autoimmune or from low GH or testosterone affecting thyroid receptor function). A dysfunctional thyroid receptor is otherwise termed "thyroid resistance." This is a critical concept. Most physicians don't get it. Some patients need more circulating T4 and T3 to surround mostly dysfunctional thyroid receptors with adequate hormone so that when the receptors are momentarily functional, they can utilize the hormone more quickly (or at all). These patients only feel better when larger than normal doses are utilized[209].

Be careful giving "supraphysiologic" doses of thyroid – you really need to watch and warn these patients to potential side effects (jitteriness, nervousness, sleeplessness, racing heart, etc.). Be patient oriented and check their extremities for cold digits.

Insomnia

Why the horrible insomnia? This is the most common complaint I hear. The insomnia these patients have is often severe. Some patients tell me they have not slept in months or years. A well-known musician recently paid a cardiologist to give him an anesthetic at night, just so he could sleep for an hour or two. I guess he had a growth hormone deficiency and the terrible insomnia that comes with it, but like so many, was never diagnosed properly.

Insomnia is mostly due to low HGH. Low HGH is associated with the inability to enter REM[210] and Stage IV[211] sleep – the lightest level of sleep and the deepest and most restful respectfully. Ambien® is a beneficial drug to aid in sleep relief, but only for short-term use while physicians properly work these patients up (trazadone is another option).

Usually after a week or two of treatment with proper HRT, melatonin, and somatropin, most patient's sleep improves and eventually returns to normal (melatonin has been tried by most of these patients, but it works very well with HGH).

Hair Loss

Why do many women with fibromyalgia have hair loss?

Women lose hair for a number of reasons, but the most common is *not* male pattern baldness. It is sometimes due to various vitamin absorption problems (deficiencies), but the most commonly reason is central hypothyroidism[212]. It can also be from lack of progesterone. Correct the thyroid or progesterone problem, make sure protein intake is adequate, and these women will regrow hair nicely.

Depression

Every aspect of pituitary dysfunction is associated with depression. Hypothyroidism is associated with depression[213]. Low testosterone (hypogonadism) is associated with depression (in men[214] or women[215]). Low progesterone is associated with depression and anxiety. It relaxes patients when it is higher (like a sedative)[216]. Low GH (AGHD) is associated with depression[217]. Low cortisol (hypocortisolism) is associated with depression[218].

Other Mental Issues

There's a loss of higher executive functions that usually occurs from lack of GH[219]. These higher executive functions consist of:

- Loss of short term memory
- Loss of organizational skills
- "Directionally challenged"
- Don't show up to appointments on time – can't judge time
- 3D spatial orientation issues

Proper HRT helps resolve this. I refer patients to a good neurotherapist for coping skills.

Muscle Wasting

Many of these patients have muscle wasting, called sarcopenia, which occurs when patients lose muscle mass from low GH (AGHD), low cortisol (hypocortisolism), and/or low testosterone (hypogonadism), all pituitary dysfunction[220, 221]. Treatment is replacing these anabolic hormones (after proper testing).

Palpitations and Arrhythmias or Bradycardia

Some patients have palpitations and arrhythmias – sometimes severe arrhythmias, and sometimes severe bradycardia.

The heart is a neuroendocrine organ. Lack of key hormones (testosterone, thyroid, somatropin, progesterone) can lead to surface irritability of the myocardium, causing arrhythmias. Think what would happen if you gave a normal young adult a handful of thyroid pills – their heart would race, maybe even to the point of arrhythmia. Conversely, if you took away someone's thyroid (or other hormones) their heart could do almost anything – heart rate variability (HRV), bradycardia, PVCs, or abject arrhythmias[222].

Heart rate variability is the ability of the heart to react by speeding up to stimuli. When patients have a growth hormone deficiency (GHD) you can lose HRV[223] (heart rate variability). This is the precursor to bradycardia[224] (which eventually can occur from a GHD), and of course another cause of fatigue.

Joint Problems and Joint Pain

Joint problems, osteoarthritis, dissolution of cartilage are caused by lack of testosterone[225] and GH[226]. This can and does cause osteoarthritis in major weight bearing and finer motor controlled joints (like the hands). Treatment with replacement hormones will regrow the collagen (and cartilage) in these joints[227].

Rheumatologic Disorder

Why is fibromyalgia considered a rheumatologic disorder? I believe it is because few doctors want to deal with it, and there are not enough true pituitary endocrinologists to properly diagnose and treat patients. Thank goodness for the rheumatologists who stepped in to help these ignored patients. At least they have some options for care.

Severe TMJ

I often see severe cases of TMJ with patients. They are unable to chew and have nasogastric feeding tubes (or central lines) in place. But that is the least of these women's concerns. Their other major joints are worse. Their fatigue is horrible. I've seen this in patients as young as 19 years.

What I've seen (contrary to what dentists say) is that a *lack* of GH and/or progesterone causes TMJ problems.

"We also found the targeted in vivo loss of collagen and glycosaminoglycans in TMJ discs of ovariectomized rabbits treated with beta-estradiol, relaxin, or both hormones together. *Progesterone attenuated the induction of matrix metalloproteinases (MMPs and matrix loss by relaxin and estrogen[228]).*"

Irritable Bowel Syndrome (IBS)

IBS occurs often in fibromyalgia[229][230]. It occurs because of the common demyelination of the Vagal Nerve[231] in patients with pituitary dysfunction which supplies the gut. This causes a peristalsis, pain problems, and brush-border[232] issues which can lead to what appears to be food allergies. Fix the demyelination problem and this almost always goes away.

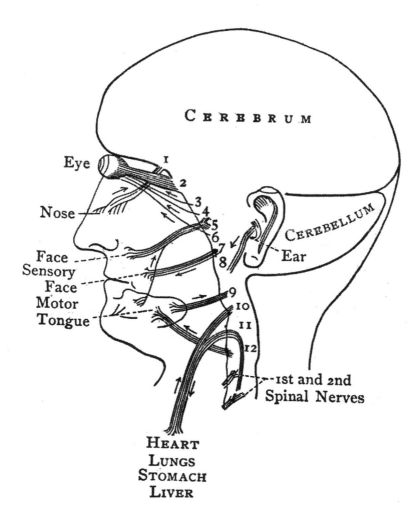

Vagus Nerve is the Tenth or Xth of the Twelve Cranial Nerves.

Gastroesophageal Reflux Disease (GERD) or gastroparesis

GERD[233] and even worse, gastroparesis, can occur because of pituitary dysfunction[234] and is fairly common in fibromyalgia patients.

Food Allergies

Food allergies are a major complaint with fibromyalgia patients. We know from pediatric food allergy studies that if the brush border[235] of the gut is not intact, then large particles of food get through, causing allergies or allergy-like symptoms.

If demyelination of the Vagal Nerve[236] occurs, then transportation problems and brush border problems develop, causing symptoms of food allergies. These symptoms will mostly resolve when pituitary hormones are properly replaced and the proper time has passed, allowing healing of the Vagal Nerve.

Demyelination Problems (Again)

Vagal Nerve demyelination is a major problem in patients with pituitary dysfunction. This demyelination is associated with (and thought to be the cause of) brush border problems in the gut (small bowel).

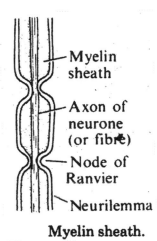

Myelin sheath.

Demyelination or loss of the myelin sheath occurs secondary to lack of key hormones such as tes, or somatropin or progesterone. Probiotics, which are simply capsules of live beneficial bacteria, help by re-colonizing bowel flora, which in turn improves gut brush border compliance[237]. Quality of the probiotic is very critical – live bacteria often must be kept refrigerated and out of sunlight – these live gut bacteria/flora are very sensitive.

Why Do Fibromyalgia Symptoms Worsen With Menopause (Surgical or Natural)?

As discussed earlier, I call post-menopausal patients with fibromyalgia "double whammy" patients because they have had years of some level of fibromyalgia symptoms and suddenly get much worse. They suffer from poorly understood and usually poorly treated (if at all) menopause symptoms. Why does this happen? Female hormones produced in the ovaries are very healing for women[238]. Proper HRT reverses this problem, but must be done with biologically identical human hormones.

Young Female Patients with Early Menopause Symptoms

Secondary ovarian insufficiency or failure[239] can occur from pituitary[240] dysfunction and can occur in fibromyalgia. Some young women and girls suddenly become amenorrheic (no more periods) and start having hot flashes, night sweats, and sometimes an increase in migraines. Either their ovaries have failed or their pituitary has failed and is no longer stimulating their ovaries. This is devastating for most young women, and must be handled very carefully. Cycling them artificially on birth control pills is not helpful, and definitely not recommended due to the side effects of BCPs. Causing someone to bleed once a month gives the illusion of normalcy but is not the same thing as ovulation.

I follow Dr. Joel Hargrove's advice, usually treating patients with a compounded sublingual human progesterone triturates of the highest quality I can find. Quality is critical, and not easy to produce. I do not cycle the patient at all. I just let them take it. Levels should be above 10 ng/ml in their blood. This almost always leads to the end of migraines, hot flashes, and night and day sweats. Maybe they don't ovulate, but at least they don't suffer as much.

Migraine Headaches

Pituitary damage leads to low FSH. This leads to low progesterone levels, which causes vascular endothelial inflammation. This leads to migraine headaches[241] and to strokes/clots[242]. Migraines headaches are not always present; I often see patients with constant moderate headaches or repetitive mold headaches. This chain of events is critical to the issue. Human or compounded progesterone is vital to achieving success with these patients.

Abnormal Uterine Bleeding (AUB)

Many women with fibromyalgia have painful periods or AUB. –The above chain reaction can fork in a different direction; pituitary damage leads to low FSH which leads to low progesterone which leads to menometrorrhagia (which is AUB). Compounded micronized progesterone (of the highest quality) treats AUB[243]. Push dose higher if it does not improve symptoms. This almost always works. Refer to ***Program 120 Handbook*** for more information.

Bladder Problems with Fibromyalgia

The Vagal nerve supplies the bladder with functionality, sensation, and autonomic control[244]. It's my contention that demyelination of the Vagal nerve, from lack of these key hormones, is the main cause of problems (pain, incontinence, etc.)[245].

Interstitial Cystitis

Interstitial cystitis syndrome (ICS) or Painful Bladder Syndrome is a condition that results in recurring discomfort or pain in the bladder and the surrounding pelvic region. The symptoms vary from case to case, and even in the same individual. People may experience mild discomfort, pressure, tenderness, or intense pain in the bladder and pelvic area. Symptoms may include an urgent need to urinate, a frequent need to urinate, or a combination of these symptoms. Pain may change in intensity as the bladder fills with urine or as it empties. Women's symptoms often get worse during menstruation. They may sometimes experience pain during vaginal intercourse.

Because ICS varies in symptoms and severity, most researchers believe it is not one, but several diseases. In recent years scientists have started to use the terms bladder pain syndrome (BPS) or painful bladder syndrome (PBS) to describe cases with painful urinary symptoms that may not meet the strictest definition of ICS. The term ICS/PBS includes all cases of urinary pain that can't be attributed to other causes, such as infection or urinary stones. The term interstitial cystitis, or ICS, is used alone when describing cases that meet all of the ICS criteria established by the National Institute of Diabetes and Digestive and Kidney Diseases (NIDDK)[246].

Interstitial cystits, from my experience, is from pituitary dysfunction. I've seen urinary frequencies drop from 75-

Program 120® Team

100 times a day to 10-15 times a day in our clinics. Most of these patients also have fibromyalgia.

Diagnostic Criteria for Interstitial Cystitis (from The National Institute of Diabetes and Digestive and Kidney Diseases Consensus Criteria for the Diagnosis of Interstitial Cystitis[247])

To be diagnosed with interstitial cystitis, patients must have either:

Glomerulations on cystoscopic examination or a classic Hunner's ulcer

and either:

Pain associated with the bladder or urinary urgency

An examination for glomerulations should be undertaken after distention of

the bladder under anesthesia to 80–100 cm of water pressure for 1–2 minutes.

The bladder may be distended up to two times before evaluation.

The glomerulations must:

Be diffuse—present in at least 3 quadrants of the bladder

Be present at a rate of at least 10 glomerulations per quadrant

Not be along the path of the cystoscope (to eliminate artifact from contact instrumentation).

The presence of any one of the following criteria excludes the diagnosis of interstitial cystitis:

1. Bladder capacity of greater than 350 cc on awake cystometry using either a gas or liquid filling medium
2. Absence of an intense urge to void with the bladder filled to 100 cc of gas or 150 cc of water during cystometry, using a fill rate of 30–100 cc/min
3. The demonstration of phasic involuntary bladder contractions on cystometry using the fill rate described above
4. Duration of symptoms less than 9 months
5. Absence of nocturia
6. Symptoms relieved by antimicrobials, urinary antiseptics, anticholinergics, or antispasmodics
7. A frequency of urination, while awake, of less than 8 times per day
8. A diagnosis of bacterial cystitis or prostatitis within a 3-month period
9. Bladder or ureteral calculi
10. Active genital herpes
11. Uterine, cervical, vaginal, or urethral cancer
12. Urethral diverticulum
13. Cyclophosphamide or any type of chemical cystitis
14. Tuberculous cystitis
15. Radiation cystitis
16. Benign or malignant bladder tumors
17. Vaginitis

18. Age less than 18 years

The Overwhelming Feelings of Weakness

Low testosterone (hypogonadism) is associated with feelings of weakness[248]. Low HGH (GHD) is associated with feelings of weakness[249]. Hypocortisolism (Addison's disease) is associated with weakness[250]. Is there surprise that there is weakness associated with fibromyalgia caused by pituitary dysfunction? I'd argue no.

Plantar / Palmar Fasciitis (Sore Feet and Hands)

Microscopic tears in the fascia of the feet and hands which won't heal (due to lack of GH and testosterone secondary to HPA dysfunction[251]) cause a chronic inflammatory fasciitis in fibromyalgia[252].

Proper treatment of the pituitary dysfunction is the most beneficial, along with time. If these aren't helping fast enough, find a physical therapist to properly use non-invasive Augmented Soft Tissue Mobilization (ASTYM)[253] to treat these problems more quickly. ASTYM is a little painful (they use a smooth-edged glass-like blade to scrape the tendon knots) but the results are promising and the pain subsides quickly. There's a caveat – whoever performs the ASTYM has to be very experienced (and completely merciless as *this is painful*) otherwise it will not work well.

Myofascial Pain

"Myofascial pain syndrome is characterized by painful, tender areas in the muscles. It is a localized disorder without any systemic manifestations. It commonly affects the axial muscles. In contrast to the widespread pain of fibromyalgia, the pain in myofascial pain syndrome arises from trigger points in individual muscles. On examination, the presence of trigger points is characteristic of myofascial pain syndrome[254]."

This pain tends to be severe, more than any injury would indicate. This is thought to be both a "local and referred pain pattern induced from active myofascial trigger points *[MTrPs]* bilaterally in the ... muscle *[which]* were similar to the ongoing pain pattern in the neck and shoulder region in FMS. In conclusion, active MTrPs bilaterally in the upper trapezius muscle contribute to the neck and shoulder pain in FMS. Active MTrPs may serve as one of the sources of noxious input leading to the sensitization of spinal and supraspinal pain pathways in FMS.[255]"

Numbness and Tingling in Feet and Fingers

Tingling comes from the nerve demyelination[256] which occurs first in the fine nerves of the hands and feet. The nerve demyelination is from the lack of testosterone, progesterone, and somatropin (HGH).

Women with Fibromyalgia have Increased Risk of Breast Cancer

Low HGH (AGHD) is associated with increased risk of breast cancer.[257] Low thyroid (hypothyroidism) is associated with increased risk of breast cancer.[258] Low progesterone[259] (from low FSH) is associated with increased risk of breast cancer (and these patients have increased migraines[260] as well). Altogether fibromyalgia patients have a heightened risk of breast cancer.

Increased Risk of Heart Attack or Stroke

Low HGH, low testosterone, low progesterone and low thyroid all cause increased vascular inflammation[261] and increase the risk of a stroke or heart attack (coronary artery disease or CAD). This must be aggressively guarded against with aspirin, proper statins, a minimum of 2,500 mgm a day of DHA and EPA (from Omega-3s in fish oil), etc. Refer to the textbook on proactive preventive medicine; *Program 120 – A Physician's Handbook on Proactive Preventive Medicine* which covers these issues in a comprehensive and detailed manner.

Chapter 7
Male Fibromyalgia

Why Do So Few Men Have Fibromyalgia?

With the onset of pituitary dysfunction (for whatever reason), and as we've said earlier, most men develop vascular problems and die much sooner rather than later.

Chapter 8
Proper Diagnosis of Fibromyalgia (As Pituitary Dysfunction) – For Physicians

Take a Good History

A good history should always come first. An accurate history is critical. Ask the right questions, spend as much time as necessary, and charge accordingly. No insurance pays for all this cognitive work. It can take hours to discover the root cause. This leads to the correct diagnosis, so do it. Don't go just halfway. My hand is never on the door.

Defining the Sentinel Event

These are causes I've seen for pituitary damage. Importantly, these are often also listed as sentinel events in the causation of fibromyalgia and chronic fatigue syndrome.Sheehan Syndrome – Traumatic or Hemorrhagic Deliveries

- MVA – Motor Vehicle Accident
- TBI
- Stressful Events
- Hypovolemic Events
- Sexual Abuse
- Concussions
- Sports Injuries
- Whiplash

Real Fibromyalgia Rx – A Pituitary Perspective

Other questions to ask:

How tall was your mother? How tall are you? (This allows you to further pin down the sentinel event – if patient is taller than their mother then it usually happened after childhood).

If You Can't Determine a Sentinel Event

If you can't pinpoint a sentinel event, you've got to dig deeper. If you don't, you might miss a pituitary tumor. Micro- or macroadenomas are rare but do occur; I find about two a year. The most common kind of pituitary micro/macroadenoma is prolactinoma. If there is no clear-cut sentinel event, and it's clear they have pituitary damage, get diagnostic studies such as MRIs.

Proper MRIs and Adenomas

The pituitary is the size of a bean and hard to examine. It is so small that even the newest CAT scan is almost worthless. MRIs (performed with contrast to help resolution) are now the diagnostic test of choice. Preferably use the new 3T machines. 3T MRI refers to the Tesla rating. Even with the best technology it still shows little details on such a small organ. Nevertheless, it can determine if there's a pituitary tumor or not, or if the pituitary is even present (I've seen MRIs read as normal when there wasn't a pituitary present – so always look at it yourself).

Program 120® Team

Physical Examination

I look for the usual findings in a physical exam. These patients tend to have high blood pressure (due to low testosterone), torn muscles (i.e. trigger points), dry, brittle, and thinning hair (from low thyroid), very cold extremities (from low thyroid, not Raynaud's), dry eyes and mouth (low tes), or dry skin (low thyroid).

Trigger Points

Trigger Points tend to be on the back, over the inner line of the scapula and over the shoulders. Be careful because they tend to be tender.

Arrhythmias

As previously discussed, these patients tend to have a lot of arrhythmias due to lack of key hormones such as thyroid, somatropin and testosterone. Twenty-four hour Holter Monitoring is an option I often use.

Parasthesia

Parasthesia is a sensation of pricking, tingling, or creeping on the skin that has no objective cause[262]. Paresthesia is the term for numbness and tingling that occurs in skin. The parasthesia I've noted can be anywhere, but is *usually* in toes and fingers first. It is annoying, and can evolve into a burning sensation, to a painful burning, followed finally by numbness. It is from the demyelination[263] of the nerves to the extremities from lack of key hormones.

Photophobia

Photophobia means avoidance of bright light such as sunlight. This is usually due to hypogonadism (low testosterone), especially in middle aged or younger men, but it occur in women also. They often come in to the office wearing sunglasses and look as pale as vampires (from avoiding sunlight). When you normalize their testosterone levels, this usually goes away. Make sure you also give them adequate (8,000 IU) Vitamin D3.

Dry Eyes, Mouth and Vagina

Occasionally called *keratoconjunctivitis sicca* (when dry eyes are severe), this usually indicates low testosterone in women who are menopausal[264].

Sarcopenia

Sarcopenia is muscle wasting which occurs from lack of somatropin (HGH), testosterone, and progesterone (in women) and a proper diet including adequate protein.

Increased Blood Pressure (Hypertension)

High blood pressure occurs from endothelial inflammation from low testosterone stiffening arteries, thus elevating blood pressure. **If a woman is post-menopausal and has high blood pressure, then she should not have oral 17 ß-estradiol due to an 11-fold increased risk of prothrombotic mutation[265].** This gives her a much higher risk of stroke or heart attack. You can use topical or vaginal 17ß-estradiol.

"Gray outs" or Light-headedness

Check their blood pressure. If it is low, look at their cortisol production from their adrenals. There is a tiny spot on the rear of the pituitary that controls the adrenals and the cortisol output. With low cortisol, patients can either look Cushingnoid (Hypocortisolism with Cushingnoid Appearance) or frail and weak like Addison's Disease patients. If they pass out often, then it's a severe problem.

Arthritic Changes

This is from lack of estradiol[266] (in women), somatropin[267], testosterone[268], or even progesterone, which causes breakdown of the collagen in the joints. This loss of collagen leads to pain and osteoarthritis. I believe this in a younger patient, is a major sign of pituitary dysfunction[269] until proven otherwise.

Necessary Labs

Viral Panels

As I've said, this isn't really my thing, but if you have to get them you'd want to get:

"A viral panel consisting of Epstein Barr, Cytomegalic virus, herpes I, II, VI, and Para-virus should be ordered. A fourfold increase in antibody titer over normal should be considered positive for that virus[270]."

I add Lyme testing, too. Keep in mind these tests are *very expensive* and often questionable.

If positive, start anti-viral medications or see an infectious disease expert for treatment guidance.

Lab "Rules"

I see study after study, and patient after patient, where I question the way the labs were obtained and under what circumstances.

Rules on Labs – 12-24 hours (ideal) fasting

No nuts – no peanut butter the week before (contains ghrelin which will give you false elevations in the IGF-1 levels)

No cantaloupe the week before

No melatonin the week before

No Provigil® or Nuvigil® the week before

No supplements at all the week before

If on tes, consider stopping it for at least 3-6 weeks (which is difficult for some patients)

Proper Lab Ranges

Program 120® Team

I see this causing a lot of problems for patients. The biggest part of the problem is the way lab "norms" are determined. All lab norms are obtained locally. That means that ranges appear to change by region. Talk to your local lab director, he or she can confirm this.

Most of these lab ranges (such as IGF-1) are determined by a formula in which the lab takes the last 1000 patients of a certain age and sex who've had that particular lab run. Then they throw out the highest 100 as abnormally high and the bottom 100 as abnormally low. The middle 800 is then considered to have a normal range. This is very inaccurate as it's usually skewed to the low end of the range and is too broad. Think about it – who requests a tes level or IGF-1? Only ill patients request these tests. This range is inaccurate as it's usually skewed low and is by far too broad.

This is a very important consideration. Physicians should confirm this with their lab directors.

You either have to know the appropriate levels for each kind of test and the equipment used, or know the general ranges that work. It is absolutely critical for you to remember that your lab may have slightly different ranges and norms. Let's give you some *roughly normal ranges*:

Laboratory Results That Gauge Inflammation

Highly Sensitive C-Reactive Protein (hs-CRP)

Normal CRP values vary from lab to lab, but normally there is no CRP detectable in the blood (less than 0.5-0.6 mg/dL)[271].

More specifically with hs-CRP, the American Heart Association (AHA) and Center for Disease Control (CDC) defined risk groups as follows[272]:

☐ Low risk   **< 1.0 mg/L**

☐ Average risk   **1.0 to 3.0** mg/L

☐ High risk above   **3.0** mg/L

If elevated, this test of general inflammation may indicate[273]:

Rheumatoid arthritis
Rheumatic fever
Cancer
Tuberculosis
Pneumococcal pneumonia
Myocardial infarction
SLE
Connective tissue disease
Bacterial, viral, fungal, or parasitic infection
Other causes of ongoing inflammation

ESR (Erythrocyte Sedimentation Rate or wESR)

Program 120® Team

C-reactive protein tests are more expensive, less widely available, and more time-consuming to perform than the ESR[274].

The ESR remains an important diagnostic criterion for only two diseases: polymyalgia rheumatica and temporal arteritis[275] but can help guide you in your evaluations and is cheaper than the hs-CRP.

Reference Ranges for the ESR in Healthy Adults

Adults Upper limit of reference range (mm/hr)

Age < 50 years
Men	<**15** mm/Hr
Women	<**20** mm/Hr

Age > 50 years
Men	<**20** mm/Hr
Women	<**30** mm/Hr

Homocysteine Levels[276]
Excellent/WNL	≤**10.5** mumol/l
Good	**10.5-13.2** mumol/l
Early CAD CHF LVH	**13.3-17.0** mumol/l
Advanced disease states (usually)	≥**17.1** mumol/l

Serum Iron and Ferritin Levels

Ferritin and iron have been found to be powerful oxidants and CVD risk factors[277]. Remember – to prevent this inflammation past age 40, have your patients assiduously

97

avoid vitamins that contain iron (and copper). This is a pro-oxidant and though you want the level to be normal, it should be at the lower end of the range.

Iron Ranges

Men	70-175 µg/dL
	0.7-1.75 g/L
Women	65-175 µg/dL
	0.65-1.65 g/L

Ferritin Ranges

Men	18-270 ng/ml or µg/L
Women	18-160 ng/ml or µg/L

Copper (Cu) Level

Usually done with a 24-hour urine test. Rarely done in adults, but more often in children to rule out Wilson's Disease. The normal range is 10 to 30 mcg/24 hr.

Mercury Levels

THg in hair seems to provide the best measure of long-term average MeHg (methylmercury) exposure (including from fish and dental fillings) and levels should be ascertained from your local lab[278].

DMPS (2, 3-Dimercaptopropane-1-Sulphonate), given orally, is the chelation treatment of choice[279] when you feel or suspect a significant mercury toxicity issue especially emergently[280].

Cardiovascular Specific Laboratory Tests

(8-12 Hour Fasting Tests)

Total Cholesterol Levels
High (Bad)   **>200** mg/dL
Low (Ideal)   **<200** mg/dL

LDL Cholesterol Levels
Low (Good)   **< 100** mg/dL
High (Bad)   **>100** mg/dL

Non-HDL-C
(Total Cholesterol Level - HDL-C Level = Non-HDL-C)
Usually   **<130** mg/dL

Note: When triglyceride levels are greater than 200 mg/dL, non–HDL-C level (TOTAL CHOLESTEROL LEVEL MINUS HDL-C LEVEL) becomes a secondary target, with an endpoint of 30 mg/dL higher than the corresponding LDL-C goals (Grundy, 2004).

HDL
Women
Ideal   **>60** mg/dL
Low (BAD)   **<50** mg/dL
 (Risk factor for Metabolic Syndrome)*

Men
Ideal   **>50** mg/dL
Low (BAD)   **<40** mg/dL
(Risk factor for Metabolic Syndrome)*

*The Program 120® team believes a low HDL *alone* requires a strict prescription for exercise of *at least* 60 minutes a day (usually they at the least need one hour per day of fast walking).

Triglycerides
 Normal   **<150** mg/dL
(I say <80 mg/dL)
Borderline-high   **150-199** mg/dL
High   **200-499** mg/dL
Very high   **500** mg/dL

High triglyceride levels may indicate[281]:
- Cirrhosis or (certainly NAFLD)
- Familial hyperlipoproteinemia (rare)
- Hypothyroidism
- Low protein in diet and high carbohydrates
- Poorly controlled diabetes
- Nephrotic syndrome
- Pancreatitis

However, low triglycerides may indicate[282]:
- Malabsorption syndrome (inadequate absorption of nutrients in the intestinal tract)

- Malnutrition
- Hyperthyroidism
- Low fat diet

General Disease Non-Specific Laboratory

CBC with Auto-Differential

You are looking for the obvious. Low WBC to indicate immune suppression/senescence or marrow problems, high WBC to indicate infection.

If immune senescence is a concern in addition to just a CBC with auto-differential you might want to get:

Absolute Lymphocytes	**1000-4100**/cmm
Total T Lymph- CD3	**78-2504**/cmm
Total T Lymph- CD3%	**62-88%**
Absolute CD4	**414-1579**/cmm
Absolute CD8	**162-1038**/cmm
CD4/CD8 Ratio	**1-3.6**

Note that in patients on testosterone a high RBC alone indicates an erythrocytosis which is harmless and just deserves watching.

Comprehensive Metabolic Panel

Also known as: Chem 12, SMA 12, SMA 20, SMAC (somewhat outdated terms)

Formal name: Comprehensive Metabolic Panel.

Real Fibromyalgia Rx – A Pituitary Perspective

A group of 14 specific tests.

* Glucose
* Calcium
* Albumin
* Total Protein
* Sodium
* Potassium
* CO_2 (carbon dioxide, bicarbonate)
* Chloride
* BUN (blood urea nitrogen)
* Creatinine
* ALP (alkaline phosphatase)
* ALT (alanine amino transferase, also called SGPT)
* AST (aspartate amino transferase, also called SGOT)
* Bilirubin

You are looking for the obvious – especially elevated creatinines and BUNs in otherwise healthy patients leading you to suspect CKD (chronic kidney disease).

Appropriate Hormone Replacement Therapy Laboratory Tests

Gender Non-specific

Thyroid

TSH (Thyrotropin) level
Ideal   **0.3-5.1** uIU/mL
Low   **<0.3** uIU/mL

Program 120® Team

High   >**5.1** uIU/mL

Free T3 (Triiodothyronine) level
Ideal   Close to **4.0 pg/mL** or even a little above.
Low   <**3.0** pg/mL
High   >**4.0** pg/mL

Free T4 (Thyroxine) level
Ideal   Close to **1.5 ng/mL** or even a little above.
Low   <**0.8** ng/mL
High   >**1.5** ng/mL

Tracking Human Growth Hormone Levels

IGF-1 levels – HGH levels are indirectly measured through Somatomedin-C levels or Insulin-like Growth Factor 1 levels (there are a total of 23 types of IGF levels but in this context I am only interested in the Somatomedin-C or IGF-1 levels). Serum IGF-1 levels appear to be the easiest and cheapest and best way to follow levels of HGH and show the effectiveness of your subcutaneous administration. This is generally how endocrinologists and researchers worldwide track exogenous rHGH and endogenous HGH. Remember these levels can "porpoise" (go up and down slightly or moderately) because of pulsatile release from the pituitary. Also increased exercise can elevate levels. Their general levels and trends (as you give or increase doses) can be tracked most easily and most accurately with serum IGF-1 levels.

Male IGF-1 levels:

Ideal Range:	**290-350** μg/ml
Ideal	**350** μg/ml
Low	**<290** μg/ml
High	**>350** μg/ml

Female IGF-1 levels:

Ideal Range:	**200-290** μg/ml
Ideal	**290**μg/ml
Low	**<200**μg/ml
High	**>290**μg/ml

IGFBP-3 (IGF binding protein-3)

All Adults: 2-4 mg/dL

The Insulin Tolerance Test (ITT) – Rarely Done

The insulin tolerance test (ITT) is regarded as the *gold standard* for the evaluation of pituitary ACTH and growth hormone reserve[283]. *The combined assessment* of GH and ACTH reserve in adults is best achieved by this method. As discussed in the diabetes chapter, this is based on the belief that insulin sensitivity is impaired in adults with both severe GH deficiency and GH insufficiency[284] (though this has historically been held to be from the central obesity of HGH deficient individuals it is now the Program 120® team believes it more probably stems from the insulin resistance occurring secondary to peripheral insulin receptor failure imparted from the lack of sufficient circulating HGH).

104

Program 120® Team

Test: Patients receive 0.15 IU insulin/kg body weight as an i.v. bolus into a vein after having nothing to eat or drink from midnight the previous night (fasting). Their blood sugar will soon begin to fall and should reach its lowest point 20 to 40 minutes after the injection. Warn them they may feel sweaty, drowsy, shaky, and hungry and may have trouble concentrating while their blood sugar is low. These are expected effects. The blood sugar has to fall to less than 2.2 mmol/L for the hormone production to be stimulated the current values for defining an adequate hypoglycemia are less than 40 mg/dl (2.2 mmol/liter) or less than 45 mg/dl (2.5 mmol/liter), although a cut-off as high as 50 mg/dl (2.8 mmol/liter) has been also used[285]. The symptoms are usually short-lived and people start to feel better about an hour after the insulin, as the blood sugar starts to rise.

Blood samples for glucose (sugar) and the hormones are taken every 15 minutes for the first hour and every 30 minutes for the second hour.

Blood samples for plasma ACTH, blood glucose levels, cortisol, ACTH, HGH, and plasma insulin levels can and are all obtained at this time. To estimate insulin resistance, the HOMA index was calculated by the formula: fasting plasma insulin (microinternational units per milliliter) x fasting plasma glucose (millimoles per liter)/22.5[286].

As one can imagine it's much easier to obtain IGF-1 levels and estimate from there.

MALPRACTICE WARNING: Do not perform an ITT on patients over 50 years of age or with known heart disease!

Evaluation of Hypercortisolism (Dexamethasone Suppression Test)

Among the various tests used for the detection of this abnormality (dexamethasone suppression, urinary free cortisol, ACTH levels, midnight serum or salivary cortisol concentrations, ACTH responses to CRH stimulation), the Dexamethasone Suppression Test (DST) seems to better accomplish the task of unmasking subtle abnormalities of cortisol secretion. Several versions of DST have been used: the 1-mg overnight, the 3-mg overnight and the classical 2-day low-dose DST[287].

Low-dose Corticotropin Stimulation Test

This is the test used by endocrinologists to determine the need for exogenous HGH. Rarely done in a real world clinical setting as it is very difficult to go through.

All Adults:
AM Cortisol Levels: **8-24** mcg/dL
PM Cortisol Levels: **2-17** mcg/dL

DHEAS levels -- dehydroepiandrosterone-sulfate (DHEAS) levels are assessed by radioimmunoassay.
Female:
All: **35-350** µg/dL

Program 120® Team

Age 45 -60:
Keep level around 150 μg/dL
Age >60:   **250-350** μg/dL
Males: **500-600** μg/dL

Pregnenolone Level
All Females: **400-450** ng/dL

Melatonin Level
Not checked.

General Sex Hormones and Binding Globulins

Estradiol Levels

Men
Ideal   **35-50** pg/mL
Low   **<20** pg/mL
High   **>45** pg/mL

Women:
Premenopausal: Follicular   **23-145** pg/mL
　　　　　　　　Luteal   **48-241** pg/mL
　　　　　　　　Mid-Luteal   **112-443** pg/mL
Postmenopausal (without estrogen)   **<60** pg/mL

Total Serum Testosterone
Men: **500-1100** ng/dL
Women: **15-70** ng/dL

Serum Free Testosterone*
Adults (Men and Women):   **1.0-8.5** pg/mL
Women
(Postmenopausal without estrogen therapy):   **0.6-6.7** pg/mL
*WARNING! Range can vary dramatically by lab.

% Free Testosterone
Men: **1-2.7%**
Women:
Premenopausal: **0.5-1.8%**
Postmenopausal (Without Estrogen):   **0.8-1.9%**

Dihydrotestosterone Level (DHT)
All Adults: **25-75** ng/dL

FSH (Follicle Stimulating Hormone)

FSH is often used as a gauge of ovarian reserve. Note though that FSH measurement is of little value in the assessment of women during the menopausal transition because it cannot be interpreted reliably and because, apparently, ovulatory (and, presumably, potentially fertile) cycles may occur subsequent to the observation of postmenopausal FSH levels[288].

Females:
Range   **3-20** mIU/ml
Premenopausal   **<20** mIU/ml
Postmenopausal (without estrogen)   **>15-20** mIU/ml
Males: **1-18** mIU/ml

Program 120® Team

LH(Luteinizing Hormone)
Females:
Premenopausal   **<7** mIU/ml
Postmenopausal (without estrogen)   **>7** mIU/ml
Males*:   **2-18** mIU/ml
*(Testing is only needed if testosterone level is abnormal.)

Prolactin Level
All Adults   **<24** ng/ml
Pituitary Tumor or PCOS?   **>24** ng/ml

SHBG (Sex Hormone-Binding Globulin Hormone) level

These sex hormones circulate in the bloodstream, bound mostly to SHBG and to some degree bound to albumin. Only a small fraction is unbound, or "free," and thus biologically active and able to enter a cell and activate its receptor. Thus bioavailability of sex hormones is influenced by the level of SHBG[289]. For example, of the total testosterone in the plasma of adult men, about 45 percent is bound with a high affinity to sex hormone-binding globulin (SHBG), 50 percent is loosely bound to albumin, one to two percent to cortisol-binding globulin, and less than four percent is free (not protein bound). Because it is the major high affinity testosterone binding protein, the SHBG level in plasma is a strong predictor of the total testosterone concentration in adult men[290].

109

Sex hormone-binding hormone (SHBG) is measured using a commercially available radioimmunoassay.

(Refer to your local lab range)

Usually for Females: **18-114** nmol/l

Female Specific Hormone Tests

Progesterone
Premenopausal: Follicular   **0.1-14** ng/mL
                Luteal   **3.3-25.6** ng/mL
                Mid-Luteal   **4.4-28** ng/mL

Postmenopausal (without estrogen)   **0.0-0.7** ng/mL
Goal with therapy   **15-20** ng/mL

Non-hormonal testing

BRCA (for Breast Cancer) if they meet testing requirements.

A negative result means you do not have changes in BRCA1 and BRCA2 genes. A positive result means you do have a change on one or both of the genes. Sometimes the test result is uncertain—neither positive nor negative.

Male Specific Hormone Tests

PSA (Prostate Specific Antigen)

Program 120® Team

The total PSA test and the digital rectal exam (DRE) are ordered to screen both asymptomatic and symptomatic men for prostate cancer. If the PSA is moderately elevated, the doctor may order a free PSA test to look at the ratio of free to total PSA. Since the total PSA can be elevated temporarily for a variety of reasons, you may want to order another PSA a few weeks after the first to determine if the PSA is still elevated.

Ideal <**4.0**
Low <**4.0**
High >**4.0** retest and/or check ultrasound/urologist referral.

ALWAYS check this before you start testosterone

Diabetes Laboratory Testing

Insulin Levels (rarely done)

Plasma insulin levels (immunoreactive insulin) are measured by radioimmunoassay. A fasting insulin of 10-13 generally indicates some insulin resistance, and levels above 13 indicate greater insulin resistance.

Patients with Type 2 Diabetes overproduce insulin because of insulin resistance. As a result, the pancreas keeps pumping out more and more insulin eventually causing the insulin-producing cells in the pancreas begin to burn out. Elevated insulin levels precede the actual development of Type 2 Diabetes by five to ten years.

111

Assessment of initial serum insulin levels is helpful guide to decide about the type of oral hypoglycemic agent to be used in freshly diagnosed patients to type 2 diabetes mellitus[291].

All Adults:
Ideal   **<30** microU/ml
Early Insulin Resistance   **25-30** microU/ml
High (Diabetes or Prediabetes)   **>30** microU/ml

HgB A1C (Hemoglobin A1C or Glycosylated Hemoglobin)

This lab is to test how therapy and diet is aiding the patient's glucose control and NOT to be used as a diagnostic lab for diagnosing diabetes because this value can sometimes be normal on patients with early Type 2 Diabetes. The glycosylated hemoglobin test indicates how close to normal your blood sugar levels have been during the past three months.

Ideal: **<6.5 %**[292] or **<7 %**[293 294]
(Note: 6 or less is still possible in some diabetic patients.)
Acceptable – Realistically   **8 %** or below
High: **>9.5 %**
Very High: **>13 %** (Admit?)

Remember "tight control", which involves QID finger sticks, once-weekly awakening to check a 3 a.m. finger stick, and monthly lab tests and office visits, in addition to frequent telephone contacts to assist with monitoring[295] is extremely burdensome AND expensive for your patients. On the other hand, the risk of death increases by 28 percent for each percentage point increase. Importantly, this risk does not begin at the HbA_{1c} 'goal' defined by professional organizations for patients with diabetes (i.e., 7.0 percent as determined by the American Diabetes Association [ADA], and 6.5 percent as determined by the American College of Endocrinology [ACE] and the European Association for the Study of Diabetes [EASD]). Unexpectedly in one review, the most important variable associated with bad glycemic control is younger age, not the comorbidity index or whether patients have related diseases[296].

Fasting Blood Glucose
After a minimum of 12 hours of fasting

Ideal	**<100 mg/dL**
Low/Good	**<125 mg/dL**
High	**>125 mg/dL**

Post-Prandial Glucose (PPG)

This is the newest, earliest lab number to evaluate before and after the diagnosis of Type 2 Diabetes has been made or is being considered. A casual postprandial glucose of more than 150 mg (cPPG >150 mg/dl) predicted an HbA_{1c} level $\geq$ 7.0 percent in one study, with an 80 percent positive predictive value – of diabetes[297].

113

All Adults:

Ideal	**<150** mg/dl
Low	**<150** mg/dl
High (indicative of diabetes)	**>150** mg/dl

Vitamin D Levels
Mild/Moderate vitamin D deficiency
8 to 15 ng per mL [20 to 37 nmol per L]
Severe vitamin D deficiency
 <8 ng per mL with hypocalcemia
 – occurs with hypocalcemia

Current recommendations are that patient levels be maintained above 32 ng per mL (80 nmol per L) to maximize bone health[298]. I believe these levels are too low and that the current literature supports levels above 80 ng/mL (near 100 nmol/L) for maximum protection.

Adiponectin Level

Two tests – a radioimmunoassay (Linco, St Charles, MO) that measures the multimeric form and an enzyme-linked immunosorbent assay (B-Bridge International, San Jose, CA), Circulating levels detected with either methodappear to be similar[299]. Adiponectin levels are paradoxically lower in obese than in lean humans[300].

To give you a rough idea (your lab might vary);
<12.5μg/ml is low (bad)
>13.2μg/ml is high (good)

Program 120® Team

Physical Measurements

Blood Pressure (120/80)

Evaluation of blood pressure
1. Make sure your BP sphygmomanometer is properly zeroed
2. Make sure your BP sphygmomanometer is at the level of patient's left ventricle
3. Check carefully on 3 distinctly separate occasions.
4. Check at various times (morning and at the end of the day)

BMI[301]

BMI is calculated as body weight in kilograms divided by height in meters squared.
Underweight = <18.5
Normal weight = 18.5-24.9
Overweight = 25-29.9
Obesity = BMI of 30 or greater

Pre-Exercise Testing

ECG-Gated 64-MDCT Angiography

With Program 120® I believe, if available, the 64 slice CT scan is the most preferable and a great new non-invasive way to perform "angiography" (also called ECG-Gated 64-MDCT Angiography)[302].

MALPRACTICE WARNING: Do not just get an Exercise Stress Test (EST) to screen – this won't be positive until anterior descending coronary artery is 70-80 percent occluded.

c-IMT (Carotid Artery Intima-Media Thickness)

The measurement by ultrasound of the carotid artery intima-media thickness (c-IMT), a major artery in the neck that supplies blood to the brain, is a reliable and valid noninvasive surrogate end point to assess risk of coronary artery disease (CAD) as it is related to cardiovascular risk factors, the presence and extent of coronary atherosclerosis, and occurrence of coronary events[303]. The high-resolution ultrasound imaging of these arteries, a convenient noninvasive method for evaluating carotid arterial walls, depicts two relevantfindings: increased intima-media thickness (IMT) and plaque formation[304]. This is currently the recommended pre-exercise screening test (by the AHA) instead of EST (exercise stress testing).

Uses B-mode ultrasonography.

Conversions:

39.37 Inches = 3.2808 Feet = 100 Centimeters = 1 Meter

1 Kilogram = 2.2 pounds (lbs.)

116

Program 120® Team

Comprehensive Lab Normals

hs-CRP Low risk<1.0 mg/L

ESR (Erythrocyte Sedimentation Rate)	<15-20 mm/Hr
Homocysteine Levels Excellent/WNL	≤10.5 μmol/l
Total Cholesterol Low (Ideal)	<200mg/dL
LDL Cholesterol Low (Good)	< 100 mg/dL
Non-HDL-C	<130mg/dL
HDL	>50-60mg/dL
Triglycerides Normal	<150mg/dL
Absolute Lymphocytes	1000-4100/cmm
Total T Lymph- CD3	78-2504/cmm
Total T Lymph- CD3%	62-88%
Absolute CD4	414-1579/cmm
Absolute CD8	162-1038/cmm
CD4/CD8 Ratio	1-3.6
TSH (Thyrotropin) Ideal	0.3-5.1 uIU/mL
Free T3 (Triiodothyronine) Ideal	About 4.0 pg/mL

Real Fibromyalgia Rx – A Pituitary Perspective

Free T4 (Thyroxine) Ideal	Close to 1.5 ng/mL
Male IGF-1 levels Ideal Range	290-350 μg/ml
Female IGF-1 levels Ideal Range	200-290 μg/ml
IGFBP-3 All Adults	2-4 mg/dL
AM Cortisol Levels	8-24 mcg/dL
PM Cortisol Levels	2-17 mcg/dL
DHEAS Female	35-350μg/dL
DHEAS Male	500-600μg/dL
Pregnenolone Level Females	400-450 ng/dL

Estradiol Levels

Men Ideal   35-50 pg/mL

Women
Premenopausal: Follicular   23-145 pg/mL
                Luteal   48-241 pg/mL
                Mid-Luteal   112-443 pg/mL
Postmenopausal (without estrogen)   <60 pg/mL

Total Serum Testosterone
Men   500-1100 ng/dL
Women   15-70ng/dL

Program 120® Team

Serum Free Testosterone
Adults (Men and Women): 1.0-8.5 pg/mL
Women
(Postmenopausal without estrogen therapy):0.6-6.7pg/mL

% Free Testosterone
Men: 1-2.7%
Women:
Premenopausal: 0.5-1.8%
Postmenopausal (Without Estrogen): 0.8-1.9%

DHT All Adults: 25-75ng/dL

FSH
Females: Range 3-20mIU/ml
Premenopausal <20mIU/ml
Postmenopausal (without estrogen) >15-20mIU/ml
Males: 1-18mIU/ml
LH Females:
Premenopausal < 7 mIU/ml
Postmenopausal (without estrogen) > 7 mIU/ml
Males: 2-18mIU/ml

Prolactin All Adults <24 ng/ml

SHBGFemales: 18-114 nmol/l

Progesterone
Premenopausal: Follicular 0.1-14 ng/mL
                        Luteal 3.3-25.6 ng/mL

Real Fibromyalgia Rx – A Pituitary Perspective

Mid-Luteal	4.4-28 ng/mL
Postmenopausal (without estrogen)	0.0-0.7 ng/mL

BRCA — Negative

PSA — <4.0

Insulin Levels All Adults<30 microU/ml

HgB A1C Ideal — <6.5 % or <7 %

Fasting Blood Glucose Ideal — <100 mg/dL

PostPrandial Glucose All Adults Ideal — <150 mg/dl

Adiponectin (Good) — >13.2 μg/ml is high

Blood Pressure — 120/80

BMI (Kg/m2) Normal weight — 18.5-24.9

c-IMT — Low Risk

Provocative/Stimulation Testing

First, you must find and befriend a real pituitary endocrinologist.

This testing needs to be performed by someone who knows what they're doing. There are risks to an ITT (see below) – seizure or even a heart attack. It is contraindicated (not a hard contraindication though) in patients who are 50 or older.

Program 120® Team

There are not enough endocrinologists. Though most are caring, kind, knowledgeable professionals, they are "below the neck" endocrinologists and have inadequate training in pituitary (above the neck) endocrinology. Here lies the problem. They can be hard to find, but you must find one.

If you find one, send them chocolate, movie tickets, and Christmas cards. Don't violate Stark but you get the idea. That's how important they are.

Insulin Tolerance Testing (ITT)

ITT is the gold standard for GH deficiency[305].

Patient goes in fasting.

I.V. line is started.

They are given 10 units regular insulin I.V. (other forms are now being used).

Goal is to drop blood sugar below 40

If they don't have an MI or seize (or die), then blood samples for GH and matching glucose levels are pulled, spun, and frozen on dry ice.

These need to be taken almost immediately to the lab.

Test lasts at least four hours

Contraindicated in anyone over 50 (due to risk of seizures or MI) unless they really want to have it and you feel like they can tolerate it.

Any peak result below 5.0 is abnormal and should be treated – whether mild, moderate, or severe GHD, it should be treated.

A delayed response is abnormal too.

Other Pituitary Challenge Testing That Can Be Done

THRH

LHRH

Clonidine tests

Exercise tests

Others

These stim tests are hard on these patients. That's why insurance requires them. Even if they fail one of these, the insurance may deny the medications. You've been warned – warn your patients.

If I suspect a low IGF-1 yet get a high one?

Retest. Retest. Retest.

Tell them they have to stop ALL supplements (you'll find they're taking tons to feel better or to just "stay alive").

Program 120® Team

If you suspect it, keep testing. Make them fast 24 hours.

When I say stop all supplements, I mean ALL SUPPLEMENTS and VITAMINS. Threaten them, plead with them. No nuts, flax seed oil, peanut butter, Provigil®, L-arginine, (so no amino acid or protein supplements), melatonin, or cantaloupe – all will falsely elevate IGF-1 levels.

And remember, if they are young (<32) their levels of IGF-1 would be above or closer to 300 not below! It's a vaguely age related sliding scale. For example a 19-year-old patient had an IGF-1 of 225. This is not normal. IGF-1 should be 400-600 at this age.

Latent Central Hypothyroidism with Thyroid Resistance

This is usually worse than it looks due to thyroid resistance. Thyroid resistance usually equals thyroid receptor dysfunction due to low tes and low GH. Thyroid resistance has been known since the 1930s (see PubMed), but has been forgotten since the 1960's. Due to thyroid resistance, these patients need a lot more thyroid than normal humans – usually 3-4 grains a day – to feel "normal." Start low and go slow. This completely freaks out regular endocrinologists and most doctors and pharmacists, so be cautious and careful.

- 24 hr Holter Monitoring

- Stress Echo – be careful most cardiologists are hacks with this procedure. Find the best, talk to them and watch the study.
- PET scan of Heart (Cedars-Sinai)
- Occasionally Sleep Studies

Other Labs for Fibromyalgia

I often get a Comprehensive Intracellular Micronutrient Panel from Spectracell™ in Texas. Go to their website for details (www.spectracell.com). This test is awesome. It covers me in case I miss something like a vitamin deficiency. They are the only ones who do it (that I know about).

Food Testing

"Multi-pathway complement antigen testing completes the laboratory workup for your patient. The immune system is in overdrive attempting to rid itself of the virus but is unable to get the job done. Every patient I see with chronic fatigue and fibromyalgia has food sensitivities. Tests for delayed food sensitivities must always be done. A RAST test for IgE allergy is effective for immediate reactions, but rarely pinpoints the food sensitivities that are identified by the complement antigen test[306]."

Program 120® Team

Chapter 9
Proper Therapy of Fibromyalgia

Let me clarify at this point that I am not a naturopath nor am I a homeopath. I believe western medicine, when properly and considerately practiced, is best. But I also believe that biologically identical human hormones are the safest and the most beneficial. Medical literature supports this. I discovered this when working on *Program120®️ Handbook on Proactive Preventive Medicine* and also see it in the pituitary research I do.

Human progesterone (P4) is completely beneficial in every regard, while the synthetics (i.e. MPA, etc.) have been highly and adequately associated with breast cancer, strokes, and heart attacks (via endothelial inflammation of the vasculature). I challenge anyone to show me differently and to adequately defend the point. I do this in seminars and educational forays, and have never been challenged (by someone who isn't drunk or completely confused, needing to increase their Seroquel®️). Until proven otherwise, I continue to assume that I am correct.

Articles that support these contentions:

Let's start with a key article:

"Natural progesterone, but not medroxyprogesterone acetate, enhances the beneficial effect of estrogen on exercise-induced myocardial ischemia in postmenopausal women[307]."

126

Progesterone and estradiol reduce foam cell formation and is atheroprotective for women[308]. *[Human progesterone (P4) and human 17β-Estradiol, not synthetics – Author.]*

Synthetic progestagens (in birth control pills for example) are associated with breast cancer[309]. *[This is why I don't ever use BCPs – Author.]*

"Oral micronized progesterone has a more favorable effect on risk biomarkers for postmenopausal breast cancer than medroxyprogesterone acetate[310]."

MPA causes breast cancer, while progesterone does not[311].

Micronized progesterone helps postmenopausal migraine headaches[312].

This is why I suggest the therapies I prefer; they work, they cause no harm (unlike the alternatives), and the patient's (previously often awful) quality of life issues improve dramatically with these treatment options.

Temporary Therapies Which Work Until You Figure Things Out

Prescription medications can keep you sane and alive until you get help. These are useful, but only for the short-term until you can figure out your patient's pituitary dysfunction and damage issues and get them resolved.

Real Fibromyalgia Rx – A Pituitary Perspective

Cymbalta®(duloxetine HCl)

From the www.cymbalta.com website:

Cymbalta® is indicated for the treatment of major depressive disorder (MDD). The efficacy of Cymbalta® was established in four short-term and one maintenance trial in adults.

Cymbalta® is indicated for the treatment of generalized anxiety disorder (GAD). The efficacy of Cymbalta® was established in three short-term and one maintenance trial in adults.

Cymbalta® is indicated for the management of diabetic peripheral neuropathic pain and fibromyalgia."

Lyrica®

Taken off of the Lyrica® website[313] – [bold and italics added by this author]

How LYRICA® Is Thought to Work

LYRICA®(pregabalin) capsules CV is believed to work within your body to calm the damaged or over-excited nerves that cause pain. *Although the exact mechanism of action is unknown, results from animal studies suggest that LYRICA is believed to work by reducing the number of "extra" electrical signals that are sent out from damaged or over-excited nerves.*

Program 120® Team

LYRICA® is a medicine approved by the U.S. Food and Drug Administration (FDA). It is useful in treating four conditions. LYRICA® may reduce the stabbing, burning, and shooting symptoms of Diabetic Nerve Pain or Pain after Shingles. LYRICA® treats muscle pain associated with Fibromyalgia. LYRICA® also helps to treat partial onset seizures in adults with epilepsy who take one or more drugs for seizures."

It's critical to know that the exact way pregabalin works is unknown. This drug appears to alleviate some symptoms of fibromyalgia and is useful to have in your armamentarium if only for short-term use until you can figure out your patient's pituitary dysfunction and damage issues and get them resolved.

Side effect of average 80 lb weight gain. This is anecdotal but appears real.

Ambien CR® (zolpidem tartrate controlled release) for insomnia issues – for patients who are desperate for some semblance of sleep until you get them evaluated. DEA scheduled. Mildly to moderately addicting – use only as a last resort and only for a short time. Keep in mind that nothing but actual treatment of their pituitary dysfunction and GHD will truly work, while using zolpidem adds only limited benefits in persistent insomnia[314].

Provigil® and Nuvigil® are medications that help with alertness and energy[315] but eventually their efficacy wears off.

Real Fibromyalgia Rx – A Pituitary Perspective

From www.provigil.com:

"PROVIGIL is a prescription medicine used to improve wakefulness in adults who experience excessive sleepiness (ES) due to one of the following diagnosed sleep disorders: obstructive sleep apnea (OSA), shift work sleep disorder, also known as shift work disorder, or narcolepsy."

In my (very limited) experience, almost anyone who has to survive on these usually has a rather significant pituitary dysfunction[316] problem, especially with AGHD. I also believe, from clinical experiences I have had, that these cause a drastic "last ditch" emptying of the pituitary of any and all hormones present. This is at least partially how they function. This incessant draining of the pituitary of its last dregs of hormones is why the efficacy eventually wears off. Again, these are very helpful medications while you try to figure these patients out, but because of their pituitary actions they obscure testing results. I require patients to be off of them at least seven days before I get original baseline labs.

Anti-depressants, mainly SSRIs (fluoxetine, etc.), are wonderful medications and work by inhibiting serotonin reuptake by nerve endings. Be aware when testing as some can cause false elevation (or even suppression) of pituitary hormones[317].

Narcotics – use them when you have to, but as these patients normalize they will have to consider coming off of them.

Program 120® Team

Stop none of these medications until the patient's symptoms have dramatically improved. Then do so very slowly. You may have to hold Provigil® and Nuvigil® for lab testing in the short term.

Trigger point injections, I believe, are occasionally beneficial but are usually not advisable to properly address pituitary issues. Tackling the root pituitary issues is the best way to heal these torn muscle fibers.

I realize how desperate these patients are to obtain sleep. Propofol® to assist with sleep (even if given by a cardiologist) is clearly not advised.

Chapter 10
Proper Menopause Therapy Based on Modern Medical Literature

Proper Treatment of AUB (Abnormal Uterine Bleeding or Heavy Bleeding During a Period) and PMS (Pre-Menstrual or Peri-Menopausal Syndrome)

I love the work of Joel Hargrove, MD at Vanderbilt University. If you're not familiar with Dr. Hargrove's work I advise you to review all of his very good articles. All of them are incredibly appropriate, even today. It's clear from Dr. Hargrove's work and the work of others that human progesterone (P4) is wonderful and will shut down most undesirable bleeding so many women (with or without fibromyalgia) suffer through on a monthly basis.

Synthetics progestins and progestational agents have been touted for years:

"Long-term progestin-only contraceptives result in reduced endometrial blood flow and oxidative stress[318]."

"The levonorgestrel releasing intra uterine device is an effective treatment for dysfunctional uterine bleeding. No difference in quality of life was observed in patients treated with a levonorgestrel releasing intra uterine device as compared to hysterectomy[319]."

These now have known side effects and increase cancer risks in an unacceptable manner, while human progesterone will shut down bleeding without the risks:

"In last years, some clinical studies on HRT users have shown that androgenic progestin- or MPA-based formulations are associated with an increased breast cancer incidence, whereas micronized progesterone- or dydrogesterone-based formulations are not[320]."

"These findings suggest that oral micronized progesterone has a more favorable effect on risk biomarkers for postmenopausal breast cancer than medroxyprogesterone acetate[321]."

Chapter 11
Vitamins and Nutraceuticals that Help Fibromyalgia

Vitamin D3

It's hard to say whether a low Vitamin D3 level is somehow the cause of fibromyalgia[322] and chronic fatigue syndrome, or that it is just highly associated with these diseases. Patients feel so miserable that they often avoid sunlight, going outside, and eating properly, thus engendering hypovitamin D problems.

Know that Vitamin D is not just a vitamin, but is also a steroid hormone that increases strength and healing[323].

Realistically, 25(OH)D levels should be close to 100 ng/mL if you want to optimize your patient's levels and health when taking Vitamin D3. I advise doses up to 10,000 IU per day of liquid Vitamin D3. Toxicity occurs usually above 105 ng/mL.

Vitamin E

Patients with fibromyalgia usually have very low levels of anti-oxidant vitamins such as Vitamin E[324]. These lower levels are also associated with higher levels of pain[325]. In reality, this may be a cheap though modest alleviation for fibro patient's intense pain.

Selenium

Selenium is a mineral. It helps in many ways. In fibromyalgia patients (really pituitary dysfunction patients) it mainly helps the 5☐-deiodinase enzyme[326] (a selenozyme) in converting T4 to T3 (thyroxine to tri-iodothyronine). It is also a critical element in thyroid receptor function,[327] which is very helpful in these patients.

Fish Oil

The DHA and EPA (omega 3s) in fish oil appear to help with neuropathic pain by helping the nerves maintain their outside or myelin sheath[328] or to heal the myelin sheath to allow the nerve to function.

To achieve a proper dose, I advise patients to read the back of the bottle (not the front) where the DHA and EPA amounts per capsule are listed. Their goal should be eventually to reach 2,500 mg per day of EPA+DHA. If they are very ill with IBS and gastroparesis, it may take a while. This will also protect at-risk patients from heart attacks and strokes[329].

CoEnzyme Q10

CoQ10 acts as a potent anti-oxidant in fibromyalgia patients and benefits them hugely. "Higher levels of reactive oxygen species (ROS) production was observed in mononuclear cells from FM patients compared to control, and a significant decrease was induced by the presence of CoQ(10)[330]." Some fibromyalgia patients report as much as

64 percent improvement in symptoms in one study[331]. It's critical that when you purchase CoQ10 that it is "natural" and "Japanese" (better quality). A lot of the other CoQ10 doesn't meet the quality of the "Japanese natural" CoQ10. Look at MedQuest's site www.mqrx.com or Dr. Stephen Sinatra's site for good CoQ10.

Ferritin

Normalizing ferritin levels helps fibromyalgia patients. One study showed that having a serum ferritin level <50 ng/ml caused a 6.5-fold increased risk for fibromyalgia[332]."

Essential Oils

I've noticed that a lot of the pituitary and fibro patients I see are using essential oils topically to get relief. You notice the minute you enter the examination room. These patients use oils to gain some joint and muscular relief, plus, essential oils usually smell great and are very soothing (seemingly more to women than men).

Essential oils can be "specially formulated to relieve muscle soreness and tension. Peppermint, wintergreen, copal, and Palo Santo essential oils, as well as others, play an integral part in this blend. Peppermint essential oil, Menthe piperita, is one of the most highly regarded herbs for soothing stomach discomfort[333]."

For full disclosure, and because of my preventive medicine textbook and work with fibromyalgia patients, you should know that I've been asked to design products for fibromyalgia and menopause sufferers (I've designed a topical progesterone in essential oil and vitamin E) by a company who I consider to be the best essential oil company in the market. Young Living Essential Oils and Gary Young, ND has been a leader in the area of natural treatments for menopause, fibromyalgia, and other diseases. Though I am western in my medical approach, I realize that some patients prefer (sometimes exclusively) these approaches. Many have been misdiagnosed and mishandled by western medicine. If you are looking for more natural soothing relief of your pain and other problems, it's a company worth checking out.

Proper Treatment of Pituitary Dysfunction (and Fibromyalgia)

Every patient is a snowflake. Every patient is slightly different (genetics, gender, age, location, extent of damage, etc.) and must be approached as an individual.

Permanent

Unless it has been less than five years since your sentinel damaging event, your pituitary damage is more or less permanent. If it has been less than five years, and if you're lucky, you may recover some functionality of your pituitary. After five years you need to get properly assessed and treated.

Tincture of Time Critical to the Process

Time for this to work is necessary. I usually advise patients that within 18 months they should have things pretty much under control. I tell them to be patient – it takes time to heal. They can get discouraged. Remember to start low and go very slow with some of these patients, and great results will follow.

Program 120® Team

Chapter 12
Proper Replacement Hormones

Most hormone medications have improved in the last few years and are more or less identical to your own hormones. Some of them are identical (and for those into natural treatments, these are pretty darn natural).

Sex Hormones

β-HCG (β-Human Chorionic Gonadotropin)

β-Human Chorionic Gonadotropin (β-HCG) is produced in women who are pregnant in the placenta, but men and women also make some β-HCG in the stalks of their pituitaries. When you look at it under an electron microscope, is made of "arms" which consist of mostly LH, some FSH, and a few TSH. This is why it's called "gonadotropin," because it has a tropic, or positive effect on gonads (in men and women) causing an elevation in testosterone levels.

Keep in mind: β-HCG is FDA approved to replace luteinizing hormone (LH) in hypogonadotrophic hypogonadism, to cause androgen stimulation (stimulation of gonads to produce testosterone).

It does not cause sterility in young patients, so I use it first versus a topical testosterone. It works extremely well in most young people (and girls). I have several men 50 years and older who do well on it. It works according to how well the gonads still function. Taking an amino acid, L-Arginine, up to 4,000 mg a day, can also give the gonads a base protein with which to build testosterone and sperm[334]. It benefits the heart and blood vessels too.

Testosterone Cream or Gel

Testosterone given as a cream or gel topically is usually the best way to go. Injectable testosterone temporarily (or if given long enough, permanently) sterilize[335] [336] people (men and women) and tends to cause liver problems[337]. Oral testosterone is hard on the liver (first pass effect) and increases the risk for various cancers in women (i.e. breast[338]). Topical tes is the easiest, least painful and most beneficial way to take testosterone.

The quality and micronization of the soy or yam used in the base of the tes cream or gel is CRITICAL to proper absorption (whether it's skin or gut)[339]. There are very few pharmacies that do it right. Patients should apply it to their inner arms once (women) or twice a day (men usually). It is a controlled substance, levels should be followed and wisdom used when prescribing.

Androgel® is a useful tes gel product but it is very expensive and, on some patients, not very well absorbed,

DHEA (5-Dehydroepiandrosterone)

DHEA is a hormone excreted by the adrenals and is considered a master hormone. There are a lot of articles available on the topic. Downstream it forms into sex hormones such as testosterone. It has numerous benefits and its levels in the body should be optimized. Remember if the patient has any personal risk factor of breast cancer, that DHEA when given post-menopausally is associated with an increased risk of breast cancer[340].

I give smaller doses to women, and tend to use a higher quality compounded version. Give it until the patient breaks out (a small amount), or until they start to get facial hair[341] (it goes away) but warn them it will occur. They can then take it once every two weeks.

DHEA is produced in the brain but more so in the adrenal cortex. It is a precursor to testosterone, estrogen, and progesterone, plus it acts as a neurotransmitter[342]. DHEA is secreted almost exclusively by the adrenal glands[343]. In human males, 5 to 30 percent of circulating DHEA is secreted by testes, and in women, the adrenals are the primary source. Converted to its sulfated form (DHEA-S) in peripheral and adrenal tissues, it has only limited hormonal potency. The primary form in circulation is DHEAS, which is present in higher concentrations than DHEA in human serum[344].

Dehydroepiandrosterone (DHEA) therapy, currently an OTC nutraceutical, is a little controversial due to sensationalized reports of epidemiologic studies and the over-the-counter availability of DHEA. DHEA is unique compared with other adrenal steroids because of the fluctuation in serum levels found from birth into advancing age. The lower endogenous levels of DHEA and DHEA sulfate found in advancing age have been correlated with a myriad of health conditions[345].

DHEA Increases Serum Androgen Levels

Clinical trials suggest that at least 50 mg of oral DHEA can increase serum androgen levels to within the physiologic range for adults with primary and secondary adrenal insufficiency, possibly improve sexual function, improve mood and self-esteem, and decrease fatigue and exhaustion[346]. This is because DHEA acts as a prohormone increasing the levels of androgens such as androstenedione and testosterone[347]. In non-technical terms maintaining physiologic levels of DHEA can "load the gun" in patients who are pro-hormone exhausted increasing testosterone levels in females and allowing adequate production in males who have the right supportive characteristics in place to create testosterone. *[Note these studies may support 50 mgm but read below for more realistic real-life doses of 0.5-75 mgm – Program 120®]*

Endogenous Production Declines with Age

Human DHEA and DHEA-S levels decline linearly and systematically with age and suggest the potential importance of that parameter as a biomarker of aging[348].

Program 120® Team

Levels (Measured as DHEA-S)

Before TreatmentDHEA-S LEVEL
Postmenopausal/   50-140 µg/dL
Postandropausal

Optimized
Males   500-660 µg/dL
Females   200-250 µg/dL

Benefits

Optimized levels protect against and/or help reduce:

1. Arteriosclerosis (prevents lipid peroxidation)[349].
2. Vasculopathy of coronary allografts (protects post-CABG patients)[350].
3. Death from *any* form of cardiovascular disease (according to the New England Journal of Medicine a low level of DHEA in a man over 50 is an independent risk factor[351]. Researchers increased levels to 100 µg/dL above the study levels of 140 µg/dL. There was a 36 percent reduction in mortality from *any* cause and a 48 percent reduction in CVD causes. Do not let your patients go untreated!)
4. Conditions associated with insulin resistance and hyperinsulinemia, such as obesity, hypertension, and untreated Type 2 Diabetes.[352]
5. Visceral obesity[353].

6. Autoimmune diseases such as SLE[354], Herpes, Epstein-Barr (boosts immune system), and even HIV[355].
7. Erectile dysfunction[356].
8. Osteoporosis in women and men[357].
9. Low levels of DHEA and DHEA-S are factors in increasing obesity and adiposity[358].

Optimized DHEA levels cause:

1. Improved energy levels[359]
2. Improved mood, well-being, and quality of life[360]
3. Improvement of depression[361]
4. Increased testosterone, progesterone, and estrogen levels downstream in the human body – Hormones are beneficial in the protection against CVD (avoid the Keto-7 version some pharmacists compound or you will not get these "downstream" hormonal benefits).
5. Improved insulin sensitivity, reduced diabetes symptoms and effects[362]
6. Increased abdominal fat weight loss (reducing diabetes risks)[363]
7. Improved memory[364]
8. Improved psychological well-being[365]
9. Boosting of the immune system preventing carcinogenesis[366]
10. The ability to reduce or even replace corticosteroids[367]
11. Significantly enhances bone mineral density (BMD)[368]

12. Elevates IGF-1 levels independent of any HGH levels[369]
13. Appears to facilitate wound healing[370] without the adverse effects of estrogen

14. *Seriously, will a statin do all of this? Will a TZD?*

Side Effects of Too Much DHEA

1. If levels are too high it can cause acne in men and women[371]. If this occurs reduce the dose. Some people are sensitive to even a little DHEA. If acne occurs from DHEA, you can give Z-Pack® (if they want quick clearing) and stop DHEA for few days. If they are on 10 mgm a day, go to every other day. (Spironolactone would work, but would take 6 months.)
2. Hirsutism[372] occurs in women, usually with darker skin like those of Asian or Middle Eastern decent. This occurs when DHEA-S is too high. Back the dose down.

MALPRACTICE WARNING: Do not give to anyone who's ever had sex hormone responsive cancer (prostate, breast, testicular).

DHEA Summary

1. DHEA is a prohormone. Biochemically it is the precursor to androstenedione (or "ANDRO"), so

there is no need for body builders to take that substance if they have plenty of DHEA on board.

2. Low DHEA-S levels at a premenopausal or preandropausal age (or older) indicates markedly increased risk for obesity.

3. Low levels at a premenopausal or preandropausal age (or older) indicates markedly increased risk for insulin resistance and thus Type II Diabetes.

4. Low levels at a premenopausal or preandropausal age (or older) indicates markedly increased risk for hyperlipidemia and thus heart disease or increased stroke risk.

5. Low levels at a premenopausal or preandropausal age (or older) almost always accompanies a markedly increased glucocorticoid level indicating stress (either from age or physical/psychological stress). Remember, low DHEA indicates high cortisol levels.

6. Low levels occur as we get older.

7. The age-related increase in the cortisol/DHEA ratio (secondary to both a decline in DHEA and increase in cortisol) is a *major* determinant of immunological changes observed during aging[373].

8. Low levels at an older age indicate markedly increased risk for depression and cognitive dysfunction or decline. Conversely DHEA improves cognition men[374].

9. DHEA stimulates the immune system and prevents immunosenescence.

10. If you get new acne or peach fuzz (women) on DHEA reduce your dose or stop it.
11. DHEA can help with various rheumatological disorders such as SLE.
12. If you have a patient on prednisone they can reduce or replace their dose by adding
13. DHEA[375].
14. DHEA markedly increases sexual libido and pleasure in postmenopausal women (and maybe postandropausal men).
15. DHEA is an androgenic steroid (thus the acneiform side effects) and will help build muscle.
16. Increasing your DHEA will reduce you cortisol, thus reducing the immune supressance associated with that glucocorticoid.
17. DHEA slows or stops osteoporosis in postmenopausal and premenopausal women[376].
18. Recent studies show adequate DHEA replacement may actually reduce the risk of prostate cancer becoming androgen-independent and thus more aggressive[377].

MALPRACTICE WARNING: Have patients sign a release/informed consent if they wish to take and are at high risk for breast cancer[378] or prostate cancer.

Unique Female Hormones

Progesterone (P4)

I've detailed enough about progesterone. Since I'm patient oriented I usually let them take as much as they want (within reason). Remember that levels of P4 get very high with pregnancy. Most women feel wonderful on progesterone. I use rapid dissolve triturates 200 mg, 1 to 4 a night sublingually prn peri-menopause symptoms.

Prometrium®is the prescription big pharmacy version (it really is micronized P4) and it works well. It comes in 100 or 200 mg capsules and insurance will cover it. This is a two-edged sword, since insurance also limits the amount a woman can take (usually one a night, which you'll find will not be enough for most women). It's an oral capsule which means it has a first pass effect in the liver – this increases SHBG (sex hormone binding globulin) and causes a slight increase risk of gallbladder disease.

17 β-Estradiol

17 β-Estradiol is the quintessential female hormone. Eluted by the ovaries almost continually, it keeps women's hair and skin soft, their bones intact and strong, protects their blood vessels, and (most importantly) assists in healing. See previous information on 17β-estradiol for more details and literature support. The big pharmacy version that I really like is called Estrace®. This is pure 17β-estradiol of

the highest quality (I think it's made from soy though I'm not sure).

I usually start patients on 1 mg a day Estrace®(it does come in generic).

Do not give *oral* estrogen if they are outside the "ten year window[379]" or have hypertension[380]. It puts women at too high a risk of stroke or heart attack. Also, do not give if they've had *estrogen receptor positive breast cancer*.

For patients who cannot safely take oral estrogen I often use the Vivelle Dot® which, though pricey, is easy to use. The biggest complaint I hear with patches is that they are too prone to fall off and cannot be kept track of easily. For these issues I tend to use a compounded 17 β-estradiol cream – 1 mg/gram a day topically. Most of my "topical" patients prefer this.

Thyroid Replacement Medications

L-thyroxine (T4)

L-thyroxine (T4) is excreted by your thyroid and acts as a floating reserve in your blood in case you need to form the more active form of the hormone (T3). What you mostly feel is T3. I usually start with a tiny dose of L-thyroxine (usually 50 mcg) and go up very slowly. I see a lot of thyroid resistance and I carefully evaluate each patient as I slowly elevate their doses of L-thyroxine. I look at hair loss, cold feet, cold hands and energy level. I also look for any hyperthyroid side effects – jittery feelings, insomnia, tremor, hyperreflexivity, or increased heart rate.

Tri-iodothyronine (T3)

Tri-iodothyronine (T3) is the active form of thyroid hormone. T3 is what you feel. If you have a problem making T3 from T4 (usually from low selenium), then Cytomel®might be a good option for you. Psychiatrists have used Cytomel® for decades for recalcitrant depression. Your doctor will have to make the clinical decision.

Dessicated T4/T3

Dessicated T4/T3 – also called Armour® thyroid is from pigs (that could be a problem). I'm not a huge fan because I think it has too much T3. Because a lot of my patients have heard that synthetic T4 (L-thyroxine) is "bad" or not as good as dessicated thyroid, I sometimes use this.

Always start low and elevate very slowly to avoid any potential for side effects.

Somatropin (HGH)

Somatropin (or HGH or GH) is a healing hormone. For most of my fibromyalgia patients this is an important hormone for anterior pituitary dysfunction. It's considered to be so beneficial that there are currently ongoing trials[381]. I only use it after I've referred someone for stimulation testing and they fail (or I do the stim testing myself and they fail). While I'm waiting for the stimulation testing I will occasionally start someone on a trial basis if their IGF-1 and symptoms fit, but only occasionally. I always start very low and go slow so patients don't suffer from "growing pains."

Chapter 13
Posterior Pituitary Dysfunction Hormones

Adrenal Replacement Hormones

When your pituitary is damaged, the little tiny spot that elutes ACTH on the back or posterior pituitary may be damaged. I rarely see damaged adrenals or "fatigued" adrenals – it's almost always this tiny spot on the back of the pituitary that's been damaged. Fibromyalgia patients are often found to have hypocortisolism[382] and this is often blamed as the cause – I think this is at least partially accurate.

Hydrocortisone/Prednisone – For adrenal cortisol replacement hormones I tend to use hydrocortisone or prednisone.

Florinef®

"Florinef Acetate (Fludrocortisone Acetate Tablets USP) contains fludrocortisone acetate, a synthetic adrenocortical steroid possessing very potent mineralocorticoid properties and high glucocorticoid activity; it is used only for its mineralocorticoid effects. The chemical name for fludrocortisone acetate is 9-fluoro-11β,17,21-trihydroxypregn-4-ene-3,20-dione 21-acetate.

Florinef Acetate is available for oral administration and has scored tablets providing 0.1 mg fludrocortisone acetate per tablet. Inactive ingredients: calcium phosphate, corn starch, lactose, magnesium stearate, sodium benzoate, and talc[383]."

Cortef®

"Cortef® Tablets contain hydrocortisone which is a glucocorticoid. Glucocorticoids are adrenocortical steroids, both naturally occurring and synthetic, which are readily absorbed from the gastrointestinal tract. Hydrocortisone USP is white to practically white, odorless, crystalline powder with a melting point of about 215° C. It is very slightly soluble in water and in ether; sparingly soluble in acetone and in alcohol; slightly soluble in chloroform.

The chemical name for hydrocortisone is pregn-4-ene-3,20-dione,11,17,21-trihydroxy-, (11β)-. Its molecular weight is 362.46.

Cortef® tablets are available for oral administration in three strengths: each tablet contains either 5 mg, 10 mg, or 20 mg of hydrocortisone. Inactive ingredients: calcium stearate, corn starch, lactose, mineral oil, sorbic acid, sucrose[384].

DHEA

Give a sustained release pharmaceutical grade capsule of DHEA. Study after study gives much higher doses than these while pushing levels well beyond, so don't be afraid optimize your doses and levels to get maximum benefits[385]. Men should take 50 mgm every morning and if weight is > 200 lbs give them 100 mgm every morning.

MalesDose

Every man > 40 years of age   5-100 mgm daily
(Weight >200 lbs?)   Closer to 100 mgm daily
(Some may require as little as 10 mgm per day, so reduce
the dose.)

FemalesDose

Postmenopausal &   10-15 mgm a day
< 50 years old
 Postmenopausal &   10-25 mgm a day
>50 years old

Watch for Side Effects

Cancer

Cancer is thought to be a risk with GH, but I refer you to a
wonderful review of this controversy "Acromegaly and
Cancer: Not a Problem?[386]" by Shlomo Melmed, who
wrote the book **The Pituitary**. Remember these points; low
GH leads to an increased risk of cancer (30 percent
increase) while optimized treated GH levels lead to a
decrease in cancer risk (by 30 percent) – a 60 percent
turnaround overall.

Oral Testosterone is associated with breast cancer[387] in
women, so don't ever prescribe it. DHEA when taken post-
menopausally in some women (who have a known personal
risk factor for breast cancer) will increase breast cancer
risk[388].

Insulin Resistance

Thought to be a risk with GH and *is* occasionally in the elderly, but GH tends to improve insulin resistance[389] in younger people – this is my experience.

Resistance

Usually I use this term to mean receptor dysfunction (as in insulin resistance or thyroid resistance) but here I mean an allergy to something – namely a somatropin allergy. This is very rare but is very dangerous. There is a tiny risk (one in a million?) when you take GH, but one must consider. Apparently it occurs only in patients who have had autoimmune thyroiditis.

Thyroid overdose – Jitteriness, tachycardia, anxiety, sleeplessness, hyperreflexia.

Testosterone overdose– Sweaty, morning erections that won't go away, build too much muscle too easily.

DHEA

If you take too much for too long, acne on the face and back, tiny facial hair. Stop and go to once a week or once a month if this happens.

Estradiol overdose (or dominance)[390]

Premenopausal mood swings, depression, breast swelling, fibrocystic disease, craving sweets, heavy or irregular menses, sleep disturbances (insomnia or fatigue), uterine fibroids, weight gain, fat deposition on hips and thighs, acne and skin breaks out, water retention, edema.

HGH overdose

Hands and feet feel swollen, brow grows (bad!), hands grow, knees feel swollen, hands feel like carpal tunnel syndrome has set in.

Chapter 14
Can Your Patient Be Considered Disabled From Fibromyalgia?

For a simple answer, yes, if it is bad enough, you can be considered legally disabled. For more information I refer you to an excellent article by Sangita Chakrabarty, MD, MSPH of the Occupational Medicine Department of Meharry Medical College titled, "Fibromyalgia and workers' compensation: Controversy, Problems, and injustice.[391]"

Chapter 15
Fibromyalgia Websites

www.RealFibromyalgiaRx.com – the website blog for the author of this book for this book.

www.AmIHealthy.com – a validated set of questionnaires you can take to determine if you do indeed have fibromyalgia because of pituitary damage. This is a great site with questionnaires designed to help doctors start the process of figuring out if you have pituitary dysfunction or not. Also, according to how you answer these scientifically validated questionnaires, you'll find suggestions for labs, where you can go to get these done, and how to get them to your physician (or to a physician who understands how to evaluate them).

www.PubMed.com – the government website where all of the articles presented in this book can be found (at least in abstract form).

www.aespmi.com – website for Dr. Purser's preventive medicine practice.

www.MyExpertSolutions.com – a web based radio show occasionally with Dr. Purser.

Patient Examples

A. **34-year-old female with fibromyalgia**

34-year-old white female with fibromyalgia diagnosis for three years. She also has chronic fatigue syndrome and symptoms of early menopause. Her husband is with her and complains of her lack of libido – they are a striking couple. She is on a plethora of pain meds and neuralgia meds.

Symptoms shows she has dry eyes and mouth and vagina, cold hands and feet, hair loss, very dry skin, hot flashes and night sweats (every day, all day), a chronic severe "headache almost all the time," crazy heavy periods (AUB), endometriosis, and feels exhausted constantly. She also has pain in her TMJ, hips and back, plus pain in her shoulder and hand muscles. She is almost bed ridden she tells you, and very sad and depressed. She also complains of memory loss. She has heart palpitations and swollen ankles.

History is indicative of a possible sentinel event, which was a motor vehicle accident 3 ½ years before (timing is right) when she hit her head on the windshield and had loss of consciousness. She is also taller than her mother by a couple of inches and she was a model some years in college, so it's not a childhood issue.

What would you get next?

Answer: Do a physical exam first. Examination shows muscle wasting. Cold extremities. Thinning hair (with extensions – she's trying to hide it). Trigger points in back muscles and tender feet. Order an EKG, 24 hour holter, and probably a echo stress test.

Then get the labs list and look at levels – if her IGF-1 comes back at around 200 or less this is way too low. Request she be stim tested by someone knowledgeable. Give her progesterone for her hot flashes/night sweats/headaches/endometriosis. Strongly consider starting her on a little L-thyroxine (50 mcg)(monitor her closely) too, and raise it slowly.

When she comes back a few weeks later she reports that her hot flashes/night sweats/headaches/endometriosis symptoms are all going away or are gone and that her libido has improved a little. (Then look at her husband and tell him that this is a critical time for him to be kind and understanding). She is sleeping much better and seems rested. You break the news to her that she may have difficulty getting pregnant and she cries softly. You add HCG to improve her tes levels but only a small dose every other day (150 units) subcutaneously.

You reassure her and her husband that her libido will eventually improve but not a huge amount – they have to be realistic. They are sad. You refer them to counseling.

160

B. **23-year-old female with severe fibromyalgia and bad chronic fatigue syndrome.**

College student who's single – fatigue and headaches are the most serious complaints she has. Her shoulders and hips hurt, too, and she has bad PMS. She thinks she has arthritis in her hands. Thinning hair and cold hands and feet.

Labs show a low IGF-1 (158), low progesterone (0.3), and a low tes (half where it should be). Her thyroid appears in the low normal range.

You start on HCG, progesterone and very low dose thyroid (increase slowly until hands get warm – she has central hypothyroidism with resistance – but warn her to watch for jitteriness or racing heart) – it's critical you get her thyroid level to an appropriate level, and that her hands and feet are warm. Go slow and carefully. Stim testing (ITT) shows she has a severe GH deficiency (blood sugar drops to 32, GH peaks at 0.9 – very low) and so the endocrinologist advises you to start her on 0.2 mg of Norditropin® and go up slowly, monitoring levels. In the next year she returns almost to normal without aches or pains. She meets a nice boy and they get married and move to Schenectady – her parents send you a Christmas card every year and her cousin Vera who also has fibromyalgia.

C. 54-year-old male with fibromyalgia

He first tells you he was a coal miner and that he's had fibromyalgia 18 years. You ask him if he ever got knocked out, and he said often when he was working. You ask him when was the last time. He tells you 19 years ago when a coal car hit him in the head and fractured his skull. His fibro symptoms started a few months later, but no one had ever asked him that stuff before – he's now disabled.

He can only walk a short distance, and then is exhausted. He has chest pain and edema problems if he over exerts.

Stress echo shows he has a cardiomyopathy. Labs show he has a severe anterior pituitary dysfunction causing him to have an AGHD, central hypogonadism and central hypothyroidism. His cortisol and ACTH look okay.

You handle him gently. ITT stim testing confirms he has a GHD and you treat very cautiously but in 9 months he is MUCH better and his pain is mostly resolved.

D. 19-year-old female with fibromyalgia-like symptoms

She does not yet have the fibromyalgia diagnosis, but her mother is sitting by her and says they are concerned because she's showing the symptoms. The young lady is petite and you start by asking her if she ever had been knocked out. She says "all the time." Stunned, you ask how and the mother says she was a varsity cheerleader in high school and now in college but is really having a hard time and is very fatigued. She is not doing well in school and is withdrawing from cheerleading.

Symptoms include some significant joint problems – hands and jaw ("Super TMJ"), premature ovarian failure (menopause), severe PMS, migraines all the time, frail and hurts all over. She has poorly developed muscles. Hip pain is significant too.

Exam shows all of the above. Has difficulty chewing and talking. Cold hands and feet. Fine hair. Maybe a few trigger points.

Lab shows fasting IGF-1 of 145 (low, it should be 450), low tes, and 0.2 progesterone. 25(OH)D (vitamin D3 level) is 19 (very low)

After stim testing confirms what you thought, she should improve with proper treatment. You probably cannot get her out of menopause (ovarian failure), nor can she bear children. Be gentle saying that, if ever. Will take 12-18 months to improve. At 19 she will probably need very large doses of GH (maybe 0.7 mg a day – much higher than her weight would suggest, but let the endocrinologist guide you here). Treat with HCG injectable to elevate her tes levels – 150-300 units injected subcutaneously each morning. Monitor all this carefully. I give my cell phone so they can text me with questions or concerns. She should be monitored constantly – this girl is critically ill and you better hold her hand while she returns to some normalcy.

E. 63-year-old female with fibromyalgia

Says she's had fibro for 25 years – she's a mess. On lots of pain meds and has been for a long time. Husband is present and agreeing. This is a hard case because if you treat (and you probably should), they need to know this is going to be a slow and tedious process. She can improve a lot, but will never be well again. She's broken, and you can maybe help her recover 50-70 percent at best. It will be complicated. Be careful because she may really have completely adapted to the miserable and painful lifestyle and narcotics.

Appendix A
Important Acronym Definitions

ACTH – adrenocorticotropin hormone – excreted from the rear of the pituitary – stimulates the adrenals to make cortisol.

AGHD – adult growth hormone deficiency

CRH -- Corticotropin-releasing hormone – used in stim testing of the adrenals

FMS—FM or fibromyalgia syndrome

FSH – follicle stimulating hormone

GHD – growth hormone deficiency

HCG – or called ß-HCG – beta human chorionic gonadotropin – a pituitary stalk (or more commonly) an adrenal hormones that consists, at a molecular level, of mostly LH arms and some FSH.

HGH – human growth hormone

HPA – hypothalamic-pituitary-adrenal – really stands for the pituitary

LH – luteinizing hormone

Real Fibromyalgia Rx – A Pituitary Perspective

MPA – medroxyprogesterone acetate

MTrPs -- myofascial trigger points

P4 -- 4-pregnene-3, 20-dione or natural progesterone

PCOS polycystic ovarian syndrome – a genetic disorder

TBI – traumatic brain injury

Tes or T – testosterone

TMJ –stands for "temporomandibular joint" but it really means inflammation of the temporomandibular joint.

TSH – thyroid stimulating hormone – controls the thyroid

INDEX

F

facial hair, 59, 141, 155
fasciitis, 85
fatigue, 11, 13, 24, 26, 27, 50, 67, 70, 75, 76, 89, 124, 134, 155
Fatigue, 17, 46, 70
FDA, 7, 129, 139
ferritin, 136
Ferritin, 97, 98, 136
fibrinogen, 48, 49, 61, 66
FiBroids, 51
fibrositis, 14
fish oil, 87, 135
Fish Oil, 135
Fluorinef, 152
FM, 22, 23, 135
FMS, 24, 86, 165
foam cell, 48, 57, 58, 127
Food allergies, 78
FSH, 26, 41, 52, 53, 81, 87, 108, 119, 139, 165

G

gastroparesis, 78, 135
Gemayel
    Nabil, MD, 2, 3
GERD
    Gastroesophageal Reflux Disease, 78
GH, 71, 72, 73, 74, 75, 76, 85, 87, 92, 104, 121, 123, 150, 154, 155
GHD, 75, 85, 122, 129, 165
gold standard, 10, 11, 16, 104, 121
Gonadotropin, 139

H

H1N1, 21
Hargrove
    Dr. Joel, 45, 80, 132

I

J

K

L

M

N

O

P

Program 120® Team

T

Program 120® Team

U

V

W

Y

Z

References

[1] Bennett RM. Clinical manifestations and diagnosis of fibromyalgia. Rheum Dis Clin North Am. 2009 May;35(2):215-32.

[2] Goldenberg DL. Diagnosis and differential diagnosis of fibromyalgia. Am J Med. 2009 Dec;122(12 Suppl):S14-21.

[3] Goldenberg DL. Diagnosis and differential diagnosis of fibromyalgia. Am J Med. 2009 Dec;122(12 Suppl):S14-21.

[4] Bennett RM. Clinical manifestations and diagnosis of fibromyalgia. Rheum Dis Clin North Am. 2009 May;35(2):215-32.

[5] Last full review/revision May 2008 by Joseph J. Biundo, MD. Fibromyalgia(Myofascial Pain Syndrome; Fibrositis; Fibromyositis). The Merck Manuals Online Medical Library. Available from http://www.merck.com/mmpe/sec04/ch040/ch040d.html#sec04-ch040-ch040c-822. Accessed 2009 June 22.

[6] Bennett RM. Clinical manifestations and diagnosis of fibromyalgia. Rheum Dis Clin North Am. 2009 May;35(2):215-32.

[7] From http://www.everydayhealth.com/fibromyalgia/101/fibromyalgia-diagnosis.aspx. Accessed 2010 March 20.

[8] Richards, Karen Lee. "History of Fibromyalgia" From About.com. Available at http://chronicfatigue.about.com/od/fibromyalgia/p/historyfm.htm. Accessed 2009 June 22.

[9] D Klinghardt: "Amalgam/Mercury Detox as a Treatment for Chronic Viral, Bacterial and Fungal Illnesses" J Explore! Vol 8, Number 3, 1997, Mt Vernon, WA (reprints: 206-721 3231).

[10] RM Bennett: "Emerging Concepts in the Neurobiology of Chronic Pain: Evidence of Abnormal Sensory Processing in Fibromyalgia" Journal: Mayo Clinic Proceedings, 1999, 74 (4) 385-398.

[11] MV Villarruz. Chelation therapy for atherosclerotic cardiovascular disease. Cochrane Rev Abstract. 2006; ©2006 The Cochrane Collaboration.

[12] Maniscalco BS, Taylor KA. Calcification in coronary artery disease can be reversed by EDTA-tetracycline long-term chemotherapy. Pathophysiology. 2004 Oct;11(2):95-101.

[13] Mikler J, Banovcin P, Jesenak M, Hamzikova J, Statelova D. Successful treatment of extreme acute lead intoxication. Toxicol Ind Health. 2009 Mar;25(2):137-40.

[14] Palazzi C, D'Amico E, et al. Hepatitis C virus infection in Italian patients with fibromyalgia. Clin Rheumatol. 2008 Jan;27(1):101-3.

[15] Cruz BA, Catalan-Soares B, Proietti F. Higher prevalence of fibromyalgia in patients infected with human T cell lymphotropic virus type I. J Rheumatol. 2006 Nov;33(11):2300-3.

[16] Adak B, Tekeoğlu I, et al. Fibromyalgia frequency in hepatitis B carriers. Clin Rheumatol. 2005 Jun;11(3):157-9.

[17] Daoud KF, Barkhuizen A. Rheumatic mimics and selected triggers of fibromyalgia. Curr Pain Headache Rep. 2002 Aug;6(4):284-8.

[18] Palazzi C, D'Amico E, et al. Hepatitis C virus infection in Italian patients with fibromyalgia. Clin Rheumatol. 2008 Jan;27(1):101-3.

[19] Suh DC, Park JS, Park SK, Lee HK, Chang KH. Pituitary hemorrhage as a complication of hantaviral disease. AJNR Am J Neuroradiol. 1995 Jan;16(1):175-8; discussion 179-80.

[20] Hautala T, Sironen T, et al. Hypophyseal hemorrhage and panhypopituitarism during Puumala Virus Infection: Magnetic Resonance Imaging and detection of viral antigen in the hypophysis. Clin Infect Dis. 2002 Jul 1;35(1):96-101.

[21] Crofford LJ. The hypothalamic-pituitary-adrenal stress axis in fibromyalgia and chronic fatigue syndrome. Z Rheumatol. 1998;57 Suppl 2:67-71.

[22] Neeck G, Crofford LJ. Neuroendocrine perturbations in fibromyalgia and chronic fatigue syndrome. Rheum Dis Clin North Am. 2000 Nov;26(4):989-1002.

[23] Tanriverdi F, Karaca Z, Unluhizarci K, Kelestimur F. The hypothalamo-pituitary-adrenal axis in chronic fatigue syndrome and fibromyalgia syndrome. Stress. 2007 Mar;10(1):13-25.

[24] Hayashi M, Shimohira M, et al. Sleep disturbance in children with growth hormone deficiency. Brain Dev. 1992 May;14(3):170-4.

[25] Beck U, Marquetand D. Effects of selective sleep deprivation on sleep-linked prolactin and growth hormone secretion. Arch Psychiatr Nervenkr. 1976 Dec 31;223(1):35-44.

[26] Yeo AL, Levy D, et al. Frailty and the biochemical effects of recombinant human growth hormone in women after surgery for hip fracture. Growth Horm IGF Res. 2003 Dec;13(6):361-70.

[27] Laron Z. Somatomedin-1 (recombinant insulin-like growth factor-1): clinical pharmacology and potential treatment of endocrine and metabolic disorders. BioDrugs. 1999 Jan;11(1):55-70.

[28] Franchimont P, Bassleer C. Effects of hormones and local growth factors on articular chondrocyte metabolism. J Rheumatol Suppl. 1991 Feb;27:68-70.

[29] Kenangil G, Orken DN, Ur E, Forta H, Celik M. The relation of testosterone levels with fatigue and apathy in Parkinson's disease. Clin Neurol Neurosurg. 2009 Jun;111(5):412-4.

[30] Denaro V, Ruzzini L, et al. Effect of dihydrotestosterone on cultured human tenocytes from intact supraspinatus tendon. Knee Surg Sports Traumatol Arthrosc. 2009 Oct 27.

[31] Jones TH, Saad F. The effects of testosterone on risk factors for, and the mediators of, the atherosclerotic process. Atherosclerosis. 2009 Dec;207(2):318-27.

[32] Kovacheva EL, Hikim AP, et al. Testosterone supplementation reverses sarcopenia in aging through regulation of myostatin, c-Jun NH2-terminal kinase, Notch, and Akt signaling pathways. Endocrinology. 2010 Feb;151(2):628-38.

[33] Krause DN, Duckles SP, Pelligrino DA. Influence of sex steroid hormones on cerebrovascular function. J Appl Physiol. 2006 Oct;101(4):1252-61.

[34] Perrin JS, Hervé PY, et al. Growth of white matter in the adolescent brain: role of testosterone and androgen receptor. J Neurosci. 2008 Sep 17;28(38):9519-24.

[35] Beckham JC, Krug LM, et al. The relationship of ovarian steroids, headache activity and menstrual distress: a pilot study with female migraineurs. Headache. 1992 Jun;32(6):292-7.

[36] Santoro N, Brown JR, Adel T, et al. The normal menopause transition: an overview. Maturitas. 1996;23:137-145.

[37] Thacker, HL. Update on Hormone Replacement: Sorting Out the Options for Preventing Coronary Artery Disease and Osteoporosis. Medscape General Medicine 1(1), 1999. © 1999 Medscape. Available online at www.medscape.com/viewarticle/408802.

[38] Adamopoulos DA, Koukkou EG. 'Value of FSH and inhibin-B measurements in the diagnosis of azoospermia'- A clinician's overview. Int J Androl. 2009 Aug 24.

[39] De Nicola AF, Labombarda F, et al. Progesterone neuroprotection in traumatic CNS injury and motoneuron degeneration. Front Neuroendocrinol. 2009 Jul;30(2):173-87.

[40] Koh KK, Son JW, et al. Effect of hormone replacement therapy on nitric oxide bioactivity and monocyte chemoattractant protein-1 levels. Int J Cardiol. 2001 Nov;81(1):43-50.

[41] Wiersinga WM. Do we need still more trials on T4 and T3 combination therapy in hypothyroidism? Eur J Endocrinol. 2009 Dec;161(6):955-9.

[42] Dyszkiewicz A. Finger cooling test and psychometric analysis in thyroid auxiliary diagnostics. Acta Bioeng Biomech. 2007;9(2):61-8.

[43] Artantaş S, Gül U, Kiliç A, Güler S. Skin findings in thyroid diseases. Eur J Intern Med. 2009 Mar;20(2):158-61.

[44] Wingenfeld K, Wagner D, Schmidt I, Meinlschmidt G, Hellhammer DH, Heim C. The low-dose dexamethasone suppression test in fibromyalgia. J Psychosom Res. 2007 Jan;62(1):85-91.

[45] Gaab J, Baumann S, et al. Reduced reactivity and enhanced negative feedback sensitivity of the hypothalamus-pituitary-adrenal axis in chronic whiplash-associated disorder. Pain. 2005 Dec 15;119(1-3):219-24.

[46] Tanriverdi F, Unluhizarci K, et al. Pituitary function in subjects with mild traumatic brain injury: a review of literature and proposal of a screening strategy. Pituitary. 2009 Dec 27.

[47] Kosteljanetz M, Jensen TS, Nørgård B, Lunde I, Jensen PB, Johnsen SG. Sexual and hypothalamic dysfunction in the postconcussional syndrome. Acta Neurol Scand. 1981 Mar;63(3):169-80.

[48] Bicanic IA, Meijer M, Sinnema G, van de Putte EM, Olff M. Neuroendocrine dysregulations in sexually abused children and adolescents: a systematic review. Prog Brain Res. 2008;167:303-6.

[49] Johansson A, Olsson T, et al. Hypercortisolism after stroke--partly cytokine-mediated? J Neurol Sci. 1997 Mar 20;147(1):43-7.

[50] Molitch ME. Pituitary tumours: pituitary incidentalomas. Best Pract Res Clin Endocrinol Metab. 2009 Oct;23(5):667-75.

[51] Colao A, Loche S. Prolactinomas in Children and Adolescents. Endocr Dev. 2010;17:146-159.

[52] Karaca Z, Tanriverdi F, Unluhizarci K, Kelestimur F. Pregnancy and pituitary disorders. Eur J Endocrinol. 2010 Mar;162(3):453-75.

[53] Fox HC, Hong KI, et al. Sex-specific dissociations in autonomic and HPA responses to stress and cues in alcohol-dependent patients with cocaine abuse. Alcohol Alcohol. 2009 Nov-Dec;44(6):575-85.

[54] Wan H, Gong SL, Liu SZ. Effects of low dose radiation on signal transduction of neurons in mouse hypothalamus. Biomed Environ Sci. 2001 Sep;14(3):248-55.

[55] Kumari M, Badrick E, et al. Measures of social position and cortisol secretion in an aging population: findings from the Whitehall II study. Psychosom Med. 2010 Jan;72(1):27-34.

[56] Irving RJ, Carson MN, Webb DJ, Walker BR. Peripheral vascular structure and function in men with contrasting GH levels. J Clin Endocrinol Metab. 2002 Jul;87(7):3309-14.

[57] Merz CN, Johnson BD, et al. Total estrogen time and obstructive coronary disease in women: insights from the NHLBI-sponsored

Women's Ischemia Syndrome Evaluation (WISE). J Womens Health (Larchmt). 2009 Sep;18(9):1315-22.

[58] Kuś E, Karowicz-Bilińska A. The influence of steroid sex hormones on collagen composition in post-operative wounds after long-term treatment with anticoagulants. Ginekol Pol. 2009 Nov;80(11):814-8.

[59] Xin S, Liu W, Cheng B. [Biological effects of estrogen on capillary vessel formation in wound healing] [Article in Chinese] Zhongguo Xiu Fu Chong Jian Wai Ke Za Zhi. 2009 Dec;23(12):1502-5

[60] Kuś E, Karowicz-Bilińska A. The influence of steroid sex hormones on collagen composition in post-operative wounds after long-term treatment with anticoagulants. Ginekol Pol. 2009 Nov;80(11):814-8.

[61] Hargrove, JT; Osteen, KC. An Alternative Method of Hormone Replacement Therapy Using the Natural Sex Steroids. Infertility and Reproductive Medicine Clinics of North America. Volume 6, Number 4, October 1995.

[62] Shimizu Y. [Article in Japanese] [Estrogen: estrone (E1), estradiol (E2), estriol (E3) and estetrol (E4)] Nippon Rinsho. 2005 Aug;63 Suppl 8:425-38.

[63] Hunt CM, Westerkam WR, Stave GM. Effect of age and gender on the activity of human hepatic CYP3A. Biochem Pharmacol 1992;44:275-83.

[64] Robb-Nicholson C. By the way, doctor. In the lead article about HRT use in your April issue, you didn't mention Estrace. I've taken it for several years, without any problems. But am I getting the same benefits as I would with Premarin, and are the risks similar? Harv Womens Health Watch. 2000; 8(2):8 (ISSN: 1070-910X).

[65] Apgar, B. Gallbladder Disease in Women Receiving ERT - estrogen replacement therapy - Brief Article. American Family Physician. Nov 1, 2000.

[66] Psaty, BM et al. Hormone Replacement Therapy, Prothrombotic Mutations, and the Risk of Incident Nonfatal Myocardial Infarction in Postmenopausal Women. JAMA. 2001;285:906-913.

[67] Psaty, BM et al. Hormone Replacement Therapy, Prothrombotic Mutations, and the Risk of Incident Nonfatal Myocardial Infarction in Postmenopausal Women. JAMA. 2001;285:906-913.

[68] Baker VL. Alternatives to Oral Estrogen Therapy. Obstetrics and Gynecology Clinics of North America, Vol. 21, No. 2, June 1994, pp. 271-97.

[69] Scarabin PY,et al. Differential association of oral and transdermal oestrogen-replacement therapy with venous thrombonembolism risk. The Lancet 2003; 362:428-432.

[70] Baker VL. Alternatives to Oral Estrogen Therapy. Obstetrics and Gynecology Clinics of North America, Vol. 21, No. 2, June 1994, pp. 271-97

[71] Psaty, BM et al. Hormone Replacement Therapy, Prothrombotic Mutations, and the Risk of Incident Nonfatal Myocardial Infarction in Postmenopausal Women. JAMA. 2001;285:906-913.

[72] Cobin, Rh. HRT and Cardiocascular Protection (January 2001 -- Live Event). Medical Crossfire, June 2001; Vol. 3 [6]: 139-40.

[73] Worcester S. Young, Healthy HRT Users at Low Risk for CV Event: WHI results may not apply to healthy women treating menopausal symptoms. Family Practice News, Volume 33, Issue 11, Pages 1-2 (June 2003).

[74] Dubey RK, Imthurn B, Barton M, Jackson EK. Vascular consequences of menopause and hormone therapy: importance of timing of treatment and type of estrogen. Cardiovasc Res. 2005 May 1;66(2):295-306.

[75] Hargrove JT, Eisenberg E. Menopause. Medical clinics of North America, 194 Nov; 79 (6); 1337-55.

[76] de Lignieres B, Vincens M. Differential effects of exogenous oestradiol and progesterone on mood in post-menopausal women: individual dose/effect relationship. Maturitas. 1982 Apr;4(1):67-72.

[77] Hargrove, JT; Osteen, KC. An Alternative Method of Hormone Replacement Therpay Using the Natural Sex Steroids. Infertility and Reproductive Medicine Clinics of North America. Volume 6, Number 4, October 1995.

[78] Furman RH. 1968. Are gonadal hormones (estrogens and androgens) of significance in the development of ischemic heart disease. Ann NY Sci 149:822–833.

[79] Thacker, HL. Update on Hormone Replacement: Sorting Out the Options for Preventing Coronary Artery Disease and Osteoporosis. Medscape General Medicine 1(1), 1999. © 1999 Medscape. Available online at www.medscape.com/viewarticle/408802.

[80] Thacker, HL. Update on Hormone Replacement: Sorting Out the Options for Preventing Coronary Artery Disease and Osteoporosis. Medscape General Medicine 1(1), 1999. © 1999 Medscape. Available online at www.medscape.com/viewarticle/408802.

[81] Thacker, HL. Update on Hormone Replacement: Sorting Out the Options for Preventing Coronary Artery Disease and Osteoporosis. Medscape General Medicine 1(1), 1999. © 1999 Medscape. Available online at www.medscape.com/viewarticle/408802.

[82] Thacker, HL. Update on Hormone Replacement: Sorting Out the Options for Preventing Coronary Artery Disease and Osteoporosis. Medscape General Medicine 1(1), 1999. © 1999 Medscape. Available online at www.medscape.com/viewarticle/408802.

[83] Hall G, Phillips TJ. J Am Acad Dermatol. 2005 Oct;53(4):555-68; quiz 569-72. Estrogen and skin: the effects of estrogen, menopause, and hormone replacement therapy on the skin.

[84] Hall G, Phillips TJ. J Am Acad Dermatol. 2005 Oct;53(4):555-68; quiz 569-72. Estrogen and skin: the effects of estrogen, menopause, and hormone replacement therapy on the skin.

[85] Shepherd, JE. Effects of Estrogen on Cognition, Mood, and Degenerative Brain Diseases. J Am Pharm Assoc 41(2):221-228, 2001. © 2001 American Pharmaceutical Association.

[86] Shepherd, JE. Effects of Estrogen on Cognition, Mood, and Degenerative Brain Diseases. J Am Pharm Assoc 41(2):221-228, 2001. © 2001 American Pharmaceutical Association.

[87] Shepherd, JE. Effects of Estrogen on Cognition, Mood, and Degenerative Brain Diseases. J Am Pharm Assoc 41(2):221-228, 2001. © 2001 American Pharmaceutical Association.

[88] Doren M. Hormonal replacement regimens and bleeding. Maturitas. 2000 Jan;34 Suppl 1:S17-23.

[89] Grady D, Rubin SM, Pettiti DB, et al: Hormone replacement therapy to prevent disease and prolong life in postmenopausal women. Ann Intern Med 117:1016-1017, 1992.

[90] Thacker, HL. Update on Hormone Replacement: Sorting Out the Options for Preventing Coronary Artery Disease and Osteoporosis. Medscape General Medicine 1(1), 1999. © 1999 Medscape. Available online at www.medscape.com/viewarticle/408802.

[91] Taguchi A, Sanada M, Suei Y, Ohtsuka M, Nakamoto T, Lee K, Tsuda M, Ohama K, Tanimoto K, Bollen AM. Effect of estrogen use on tooth retention, oral bone height, and oral bone porosity in Japanese postmenopausal women. Menopause. 2004 Sep-Oct;11(5):556-62.

[92] McKuen BS, Alves BS. Estrogen action in the central nervous system. *Endocrin Rev* .1999;20:279-307.

[93] Haan MN, Klein R, Klein BE, Deng Y, Blythe LK, Seddon JM, Musch DC, Kuller LH, Hyman LG, Wallace RB. Hormone therapy and age-related macular degeneration: the Women's Health Initiative Sight Exam Study. Arch Ophthalmol. 2006 Jul;124(7):988-92.

[94] Klein BEK, Klein R, Ritter LL. Is there evidence of an estrogen effect on age-related lens opacities? Arch Ophthalmol. 1994;112:85-91.

[95] Shepherd, JE. Effects of Estrogen on Cognition, Mood, and Degenerative Brain Diseases. J Am Pharm Assoc 41(2):221-228, 2001. © 2001 American Pharmaceutical Association.

[96] Doren M. Hormonal replacement regimens and bleeding. Maturitas. 2000 Jan;34 Suppl 1:S17-23.

[97] Punnonen R, Vilska S, Rauramo L. Skinfold thickness and long-term post-menopausal hormone therapy. Maturitas. 1984 Apr;5(4):259-62.

[98] Stampfer MJ, Colditz GA. Estrogen replacement and coronary heart disease: a quantitative assessment of the epidemiologic evidence. Prev Med. 1991;20:47-63.

[99] Stampfer MJ, Colditz GA, Willett WC, Manson JE, Rosner B, Speizer FE, Hennekens CH. Postmenopausal estrogen therapy and cardiovascular disease. Ten-year follow-up from the nurses' health study. N Engl J Med. 1991 Sep 12;325(11):756-62.

[100] [no author listed] NHBLI NIH NEWS. WHI Study Finds No Heart Disease Benefit, Increased Stroke Risk With Estrogen Alone. Tuesday,

April 13, 2004, 4:00 p.m. ET. [online] Available at www.nhlbi.nih.gov/whi. Accessed 2006 Oct 7.

[101] Chen H ; Chen Y ; Tian W ; Lei S ; Peng R. [Effects of estradiol and isoflavoid on the expression of adhesion molecules on neutrophils] Hua Xi Yi Ke Da Xue Xue Bao. 2001; 32(1):27-31 (ISSN: 0257-7712).

[102] Wise PM; Dubal DB; Wilson ME; Rau SW; Böttner M. Minireview: neuroprotective effects of estrogen-new insights into mechanisms of action. Endocrinology. 2001; 142(3):969-73 (ISSN: 0013-7227).

[103] Shoupe D. Hormone replacement therapy: reassessing the risks and benefits. Hosp Pract (Minneap). 1999 Aug 15;34(8):97-103, 107-8, 113-4.

[104] Shoupe D. Hormone replacement therapy: reassessing the risks and benefits. Hosp Pract (Minneap). 1999 Aug 15;34(8):97-103, 107-8, 113-4.

[105] Shoupe D. Hormone replacement therapy: reassessing the risks and benefits. Hosp Pract (Minneap). 1999 Aug 15;34(8):97-103, 107-8, 113-4.

[106] Meisler, JG. Toward Optimal Health: The Experts Provide a Current Perspective on Perimenopause. J Womens Health 12(7):609-615, 2003. © 2003 Mary Ann Liebert, Inc.

[107] Dupont WD, Page DL: Menopausal, estrogen replacement therapy, and breast cancer. Arch Intern Med 151:67-72, 1991.

[108] Effects of hormone replacement therapy on endometrial histology in postmenopausal women. The Postmenopausal Estrogen/Progestin Interventions (PEPI) Trial. The Writing Group for the PEPI Trial. JAMA. 1996;275:370-375.

[109] [no author listed] Findings from the WHI Postmenopausal Hormone Therapy Trials. Available online at www.nhlbi.nih.gov/whi/. Accessed 2006 Sep 10.

[110] Meisler, JG. Toward Optimal Health: The Experts Provide a Current Perspective on Perimenopause. J Womens Health 12(7):609-615, 2003. © 2003 Mary Ann Liebert, Inc.

[111] Prior JC, Vigna Y, Sciarretta D, et al. Conditioning exercise decreases premenstrual symptoms: a prospective, controlled 6-month trial. *Fertil Steril.* 1987;47:402-8.

[112] Wolanske, KA; Gordon, RL. Uterine Artery Embolization: Where Does it Stand in the Management of Uterine Leiomyomas? Part 2. Appl Radiol 33(10):18-25, 2004. © 2004 Anderson Publishing, Ltd.

[113] Fettes I. Migraine in the menopause. Neurology. 1999;53 (suppl 1):S29-S33.

[114] Walsh BW, Kuller LH, Wild RA, et al. Effects of raloxifene on serum lipids and coagulation factors in healthy postmenopausal women. JAMA. 1998;2790:1445-1451.

[115] Hulley S, Grady D, Bush T, et al. Randomized trial of estrogen plus progestin for secondary prevention of coronary heart disease in postmenopausal women: Heart and Estrogen/progestin Replacement Study (HERS) Research Group. JAMA 1998;280:605-613.

[116] Birkenfeld L, Yemini M, Kase NG, et al. Menopause-related oral alveolar bone resorption: a review of relatively unexplored consequences of estrogen deficiency. Menopause. 1999;6:129-133.

[117] Freeman EW, et al. Associations of hormones and menopausal status with depressed mood in women with no history of depression. Arch Gen Psychiatry April 2006;63:375-82.

[118] Campagnoli C; Colombo P; De Aloysio D; Gambacciani M; Grazioli I; Nappi C; Serra GB; Genazzani AR. Positive effects on cardiovascular and breast metabolic markers of oral estradiol and dydrogesterone in comparison with transdermal estradiol and norethisterone acetate. Maturitas. 2002; 41(4):299-311 (ISSN: 0378-5122).

[119] Bastian LA, Smith CM, Nanda K. Is this woman perimenopausal? JAMA. 2003 Feb 19;289(7):895-902.

[120] Dalal, S; Zhukovsky, DS. Pathoilable online at physiology and Management of Hot Flashes. www.SupportiveOncology.net; VOLUME 4, NUMBER 7; JULY/AUGUST 2006. Available online at www.SupportiveOncology.net.

[121] Freedman RR, Norton D, Woodward S, et al. Core body temperature and circadian rhythm of hot flashes in menopausal women. J Clin Endocrinol Metab 1995;80:2354–2358.

[122] Cho JJ, Cadet P, Salamon E, Mantione K, Stefano GB. The nongenomic protective effects of estrogen on the male cardiovascular

system: clinical and therapeutic implications in aging men. Med Sci Monit. 2003 Mar;9(3):RA63-8.

[123] Hargrove, JT; Osteen, KC. An Alternative Method of Hormone Replacement Therpay Using the Natural Sex Steroids. Infertility and Reproductive Medicine Clinics of North America. Volume 6, Number 4, October 1995.

[124] [No authors listed] Medroxyprogesterone acetate. IARC Monogr Eval Carcinog Risk Chem Hum. 1979 Dec;21:417-29.

[125] Klaiber EL; Vogel W; Rako S. A critique of the Women's Health Initiative hormone therapy study. Fertil Steril. 2005; 84(6):1589-601 (ISSN: 1556-5653).

[126] Thomas T, Rhodin J, Clark L, Garces A. Progestins initiate adverse events of menopausal estrogen therapy. Climacteric. 2003 Dec;6(4):293-301.

[127] Campagnoli C, Clavel-Chapelon F, Kaaks R, Peris C, Berrino F. Progestins and progesterone in hormone replacement therapy and the risk of breast cancer. J Steroid Biochem Mol Biol. 2005 Jul;96(2):95-108.

[128] Cushman M, Legault C, Barrett-Connor E, et al. Effect of postmenopausal hormones on inflammation-sensitive proteins: the Postmenopausal Estrogen/Progestin Interventions (PEPI) Study. Circulation. 1999;100:717-722.

[129] Clark MK, Sowers M, Levy B, Nichols S. Bone mineral density loss and recovery during 48 months in first-time users of depot medroxyprogesterone acetate. Fertil Steril. 2006 Nov;86(5):1466-74.

[130] Archer B, Irwin D, Jensen K, Johnson ME, Rorie J. Depot medroxyprogesterone. Management of side-effects commonly associated with its contraceptive use. J Nurse Midwifery. 1997 Mar-Apr;42(2):104-11.

[131] Klaiber EL; Vogel W; Rako S. A critique of the Women's Health Initiative hormone therapy study. Fertil Steril. 2005; 84(6):1589-601 (ISSN: 1556-5653).

[132] Effects of estrogen or estrogen/progestin regimens on heart disease risk factors in postmenopausal women. Writing Group for the PEPI Trial. JAMA. 1995;273:1389-96.

189

[133] Hargrove JT, Maxson WS, Wentz AC, Burnett LS. Menopausal hormone replacement therapy with continuous daily oral micronized estradiol and progesterone. Obstet Gynecol. 1989 Apr;73(4):606-12.

[134] Sitruk-Ware R, Bricaire C, DeLignieres B, et al. Oral Micronized progesterone. Bioavailability pharmacokinetics, pharmacological and therapeutic implications—A Review, Contraception. 1987; 36:373-402.

[135] WEN-SEN LEE, CHAO-WEI LIU, SHU-HUI JUAN, YU-CHIH LIANG, PEI-YIN HO, AND YI-HSUAN LEE. Molecular Mechanism of Progesterone-Induced Antiproliferation in Rat Aortic Smooth Muscle Cells. Endocrinology 144(7):2785–2790. Copyright © 2003 by The Endocrine Society doi: 10.1210/en.2003-0045.

[136] McCrohon JA; Nakhla S; Jessup W; Stanley KK; Celermajer DS. Estrogen and progesterone reduce lipid accumulation in human monocyte-derived macrophages: a sex-specific effect. Circulation. 1999; 100(23):2319-25 (ISSN: 0009-7322).

[137] Campagnoli C, Clavel-Chapelon F, aaks R, Peris C, Berrino F. Progestins and progesterone in hormone replacement therapy and the risk of breast cancer. J Steroid Biochem Mol Biol. 2005 Jul;96(2):95-108.

[138] Lydeking-Olsen E, Beck-Jensen JE, Setchell KD, Holm-Jensen T. Soymilk or progesterone for prevention of bone loss--a 2 year randomized, placebo-controlled trial. Eur J Nutr. 2004 Aug;43(4):246-57.

[139] Randall TC, Kurman RJ. Progestin treatment of atypical hyperplasia and well-differentiated carcinoma of the endometrium in women under age 40. Obstet Gynecol 1997;90:434-40.

[140] Fraser IS. Regulating menstrual bleeding. A prime function of progesterone. J Reprod Med 1999;44(2 suppl):158-64.

[141] Arafat ES, Hargrove JT, Maxson WS, Desiderio DM, Wentz AC, Andersen RN. Sedative and hypnotic effects of oral administration of micronized progesterone may be mediated through its metabolites. Am J Obstet Gynecol. 1988 Nov;159(5):1203-9.

[142] Vanselow W, Dennerstein L, Greenwood KM, de Lignieres B. Effect of progesterone and its 5 alpha and 5 beta metabolites on

symptoms of premenstrual syndrome according to route of administration. J Psychosom Obstet Gynaecol. 1996 Mar;17(1):29-38.
[143] Maxson WS. The use of progesterone in the treatment of PMS. Clin Obstet Gynecol. 1987:30:465-477
[144] Ahlgrimm, M. (May 2003). Managing pms and perimenopause symptoms The role of compounded medications, Advance for Nurse Practitioners, (11)5, p. 53.
[145] APGAR, B.S., GREENBERG, G. Practical Therapeutics Using Progestins in Clinical Practice. AFP - October 15, 2000.
[146] Fitzpatrick, LA; Pace, C; Wiita, B. Comparison of Regimens Containing Oral Micronized Progesterone or Medroxyprogesterone Acetate on Quality of Life in Postmenopausal Women: A Cross-Sectional Survey. Journal of Women's Health & Gender-Based Medicine. May 2000, Vol. 9, No. 4 :381 -387.
[147] Davis SR, Guay AT, Shifren JL, Mazer NA. Endocrine aspects of female sexual dysfunction. J Sex Med. 2004 Jul;1(1):82-6.
[148] Hargrove JT, Maxson WS, Wentz AC, Burnett LS. Menopausal hormone replacement therapy with continuous daily oral micronized estradiol and progesterone. Obstet Gynecol. 1989:73: 606-612.
[149] Kapila S, Wang W, Uston K. Matrix metalloproteinase induction by relaxin causes cartilage matrix degradation in target synovial joints. Ann N Y Acad Sci. 2009 Apr;1160:322-8.
[150] Voumvourakis KI, Tsiodras S, Kitsos DK, Stamboulis E. Gender hormones: role in the pathogenesis of central nervous system disease and demyelination. Curr Neurovasc Res. 2008 Nov;5(4):224-35.
[151] Zumpe D, Clancy AN, Michael RP. Progesterone decreases mating and estradiol uptake in preoptic areas of male monkeys. Physiol Behav. 2001 Nov-Dec;74(4-5):603-12.
[152] Abrams D. Use of androgens in patients who have HIV/AIDS: what we know about the effect of androgens on wasting and lipodystrophy. AIDS Read. 2001 Mar;11(3):149-56.
[153] Smith AM, Jones RD, Channer KS. The influence of sex hormones on pulmonary vascular reactivity: possible vasodilator therapies for the treatment of pulmonary hypertension. Curr Vasc Pharmacol. 2006 Jan;4(1):9-15.

[154] Golden SH, Maguire A, Ding J, Crouse JR, Cauley JA, Zacur H, Szklo M. Endogenous postmenopausal hormones and carotid atherosclerosis: a case-control study of the atherosclerosis risk in communities cohort. Am J Epidemiol. 2002 Mar 1;155(5):437-45.

[155] Dobrzycki S, Serwatka W, Nadlewski S, et al. An assessment of correlations between endogenous sex hormone levels and the extensiveness of coronary heart disease and the ejection fraction of the left ventricle in males. J Med Invest. 2003 Aug;50(3-4):162-9.

[156] Phillips GB, Pinkernell BH, Jing TY. Are major risk factors for myocardial infarction the major predictors of degree of coronary artery disease in men? Metabolism. 2004 Mar;53(3):324-9.

[157] Dzugan SA, Smith RA. Hypercholesterolemia treatment: a new hypothesis or just an accident? Med Hypothesis. 2002 Dec;59(6):751-6.

[158] Dzugan SA, Smith RA. Broad spectrum restoration in natural steroid hormones as possible treatment for hypercholesterolemia. Bull Urg Rec Med. 2002;3(2):278-84.

[159] English KM, Steeds R, Jones TH, Channer KS: Testosterone and coronary heart disease: is there a link? Q J Med 90:787–791, 1997.

[160] Anderson RA, Ludlam CA, Wu FC: Haemostatic effects of supraphysiological levels of testosterone in normal men. Thromb Haemost 74:693–697, 1995.

[161] Webb CM, McNeill JG, Hayward CS, Zeigler D, Collins P: Effects of testosterone on coronary vasomotor regulation in men with coronary heart disease. Circulation 100:1690–1696, 1999.

[162] Osuna JA, Gomez-Perez R, Arata-Bellabarba G, Villaroel V. Relationship between BMI, total testosterone, sex hormone-binding-globulin, leptin, insulin and insulin resistance in obese men. Arch Androl. 2006 Sep-Oct;52(5):355-61.

[163] Simon D, Charles MA, Nahoul K, Orssaud G, Kremski J, Hully V, Joubert E, Papoz L, Eschwege E: Association between plasma total testosterone and cardiovascular risk factors in healthy adult men: the Telecom Study. J Clin Endocrinol Metab 82:682–685, 1997.

[164] Osuna JA, Gomez-Perez R, Arata-Bellabarba G, Villaroel V. Relationship between BMI, total testosterone, sex hormone-binding-

192

globulin, leptin, insulin and insulin resistance in obese men. Arch Androl. 2006 Sep-Oct;52(5):355-61.

[165] Hogervorst E, Bandelow S, Combrinck M, Smith AD. Low free testosterone is an independent risk factor for Alzheimer's disease. Exp Gerontol. 2004 Nov-Dec;39(11-12):1633-9.

[166] Winters, SJ. Current Status of Testosterone Replacement Therapy in Men. Arch Fam Med. 1999;8:257-263.

[167] Carrier S, Zvara P, Lue TF. Erectile dysfunction. *Endocrinol Metab Clin North Am.* 1994;23:773-782.

[168] Shifren JL, Braunstein GD, Simon JA, Casson PR, Buster JE, Redmond GP, Burki RE, Ginsburg ES, Rosen RC, Leiblum SR, Caramelli KE, Mazer NA. Transdermal testosterone treatment in women with impaired sexual function after oophorectomy. N Engl J Med. 2000 Sep 7;343(10):682-8.

[169] Mooradian AD, Morley JE, Korenman SG. Biological actions of androgens. *Endocr Rev.* 1987;8:1-28.

[170] Veldhuis JD, Keenan DM, Mielke K, Miles JM, Bowers CY. Testosterone supplementation in healthy older men drives GH and IGF-I secretion without potentiating peptidyl secretagogue efficacy. Eur J Endocrinol. 2005 Oct;153(4):577-86.

[171] Yael Waknine. Testosterone Replacement Improves Exercise Capacity in Men With CHF. [online] Available on Medscape Medical News 2005. © 2005 Medscape at www.medscape.com/viewarticle/506223

[172] Malkin CJ, Pugh PJ, West JN, van Beek EJ, Jones TH, Channer KS. Testosterone therapy in men with moderate severity heart failure: a double-blind randomized placebo controlled trial. Eur Heart J. 2006 Jan;27(1):57-64.

[173] Walston, J; Hadley, EC; Ferrucci, L; Guralnik, JM; Newman, AB; Studenski, SA; Ershler, WB; Harris, T; Fried, LP. Research Agenda for Frailty in Older Adults. J Am Geriatr Soc. 2006;54(6):991-1001. ©2006 Blackwell Publishing.

[174] Hackney AC, Moore AW, Brownlee KK. Testosterone and endurance exercise: development of the "exercise-hypogonadal male condition". Acta Physiol Hung. 2005;92(2):121-37.

[175] Demling RH. The role of anabolic hormones for wound healing in catabolic States. J Burns Wounds. 2005 Jan 17;4:e2.

[176]Hardman MJ, Ashcroft GS. Hormonal influences on wound healing: a review of current experimental data. WOUNDS. 2005;17(11):313-320.

[177] Muller M; Aleman A; Grobbee DE; de Haan EH; van der Schouw YT. Endogenous sex hormone levels and cognitive function in aging men: is there an optimal level? Neurology. 2005; 64(5):866-71 (ISSN: 1526-632X).

[178] Brian C. Lund, Pharm.D., Kristine A. Bever-Stille, Pharm.D., and Paul J. Perry, Ph.D. Testosterone and Andropause: The Feasibility of Testosterone Replacement Therapy in Elderly Men. Pharmacotherapy 19(8):951-956, 1999. © 1999 Pharmacotherapy Publications.

[179] American College of Endocrinologists and American Association of Clinical Endocrinologists. *Guidelines for the Evaluation and Treatment of Male Sexual Dysfunction.* American College of Endocrinologists and American Association of Clinical Endocrinologists; 1998:4.

[180] Aversa A, Isidori AM, De Martino MU, et al. Androgens and penile erection evidence for a direct relationship between free testosterone and cavernous vasodilation in men with ED. Clin Endocrinol (Oxf). 2000;53:517-522.

[181] [Article in Chinese] Chen X, Li X, Huang HY, Li X, Lin JF. [Effects of testosterone on insulin receptor substrate-1 and glucose transporter 4 expression in cells sensitive to insulin] Zhonghua Yi Xue Za Zhi. 2006 Jun 6;86(21):1474-7.

[182] Braga-Basaria M, Dobs AS, Muller DC, Carducci MA, John M, Egan J, Basaria S. Metabolic syndrome in men with prostate cancer undergoing long-term androgen-deprivation therapy. J Clin Oncol. 2006 Aug 20;24(24):3979-83.

[183] Svartberg J. Epidemiology: testosterone and the metabolic syndrome. Int J Impot Res. 2006 Jul 20.

[184] Fogari R, Preti P, Zoppi A, Fogari E, Rinaldi A, Corradi L, Mugellini A. Serum testosterone levels and arterial blood pressure in the elderly. Hypertens Res. 2005 Aug;28(8):625-30.

[185] Huisman HW, Schutte AE, Van Rooyen JM, Malan NT, Malan L, Schutte R, Kruger A. The influence of testosterone on blood pressure and risk factors for cardiovascular disease in a black South African population. Ethn Dis. 2006 Summer;16(3):693-8.

[186] Vondracek, SF; Hansen, LB. Current Approaches to the Management of Osteoporosis in Men. Am J Health-Syst Pharm 61(17):1801-1811, 2004. © 2004 American Society of Health-System Pharmacists.

[187] Isidori AM, Giannetta E, Greco EA, Gianfrilli D, Bonifacio V, Isidori A, Lenzi A, Fabbri A. Effects of testosterone on body composition, bone metabolism and serum lipid profile in middle-aged men: a meta-analysis. Clin Endocrinol (Oxf). 2005 Sep;63(3):280-93.

[188] Reported by By Karla Gale. Testosterone May Slow Progress of MS in Men. Reuters Health Information 2006. © 2006 Reuters Ltd. [online] Available on Medscape® at www.medscape.com/viewarticle/529199.

[189] Markianos M; Panas M; Kalfakis N; Vassilopoulos D. Plasma testosterone in male patients with Huntington's disease: relations to severity of illness and dementia. Ann Neurol. 2005; 57(4):520-5 (ISSN: 0364-5134).

[190] Moffat SD. Effects of testosterone on cognitive and brain aging in elderly men. Ann N Y Acad Sci. 2005; 1055:80-92 (ISSN: 0077-8923).

[191] Bialek M, Zaremba P, Borowicz KK, Czuczwar SJ. Neuroprotective role of testosterone in the nervous system. Pol J Pharmacol. 2004 Sep-Oct;56(5):509-18.

[192] Finazzi G, Gregg XT, Barbui T, Prchal JT. Idiopathic erythrocytosis and other non-clonal polycythemias. Best Pract Res Clin Haematol. 2006;19(3):471-82.

[193] Ferrucci L, Maggio M, Bandinelli S, Basaria S, Lauretani F, Ble A, Valenti G, Ershler WB, Guralnik JM, Longo DL. Low testosterone levels and the risk of anemia in older men and women. Arch Intern Med. 2006 Jul 10;166(13):1380-8.

[194] McVary KT; McKenna KE. The relationship between erectile dysfunction and lower urinary tract symptoms: epidemiological, clinical, and basic science evidence. Curr Urol Rep. 2004; 5(4):251-7 (ISSN: 1527-2737).

[195] Kaminetsky J. Comorbid LUTS and erectile dysfunction: optimizing their management. Curr Med Res Opin. 2006 Dec;22(12):2497-506.

[196] Spector TD, Perry LA, Tubb G, Silman AJ, Huskisson EC. Low free testosterone levels in rheumatoid arthritis. Ann Rheum Dis. 1988 Jan;47(1):65-8.

[197] Cutolo M, Balleari E, Giusti M, Monachesi M, Accardo S. Sex hormone status of male patients with rheumatoid arthritis: evidence of low serum concentrations of testosterone at baseline and after human chorionic gonadotropin stimulation. Arthritis Rheum. 1988 Oct;31(10):1314-7.

[198] Rhoden EL; Morgentaler A. Testosterone replacement therapy in hypogonadal men at high risk for prostate cancer: results of 1 year of treatment in men with prostatic intraepithelial neoplasia. J Urol. 2003; 170(6 Pt 1):2348-51 (ISSN: 0022-5347)

[199] Smith AM, English KM, Malkin CJ, Jones RD, Jones TH, Channer KS. Testosterone does not adversely affect fibrinogen or tissue plasminogen activator (tPA) and plasminogen activator inhibitor-1 (PAI-1) levels in 46 men with chronic stable angina. Eur J Endocrinol. 2005 Feb;152(2):285-91.

[200] Orwoll E, Lambert LC, Marshall LM, Blank J, Barrett-Connor E, Cauley J, Ensrud K, Cummings SR; Osteoporotic Fractures in Men Study Group. Endogenous testosterone levels, physical performance, and fall risk in older men. Arch Intern Med. 2006 Oct 23;166(19):2124-31.

[201] Izquierdo-Alvarez S, Bocos-Terraz JP, et al. Is there an association between fibromyalgia and below-normal levels of urinary cortisol? BMC Res Notes. 2008 Dec 22;1:134.

[202] Calis M, Gökçe C, et al. Investigation of the hypothalamo-pituitary-adrenal axis (HPA) by 1 microg ACTH test and metyrapone test in patients with primary fibromyalgia syndrome. J Endocrinol Invest. 2004 Jan;27(1):42-6.

[203] Zargar AH, Laway BA, et al. A critical evaluation of signs and symptoms in the diagnosis of Addison's diseases. J Assoc Physicians India. 2001 May;49:523-6.

[204] Nettleship JE, Jones RD, Channer KS, Jones TH. Testosterone and coronary artery disease. Front Horm Res. 2009;37:91-107.

[205] Belmont A, Agar N, Hugeron C, Gallais B, Azouvi P. Fatigue and traumatic brain injury. Ann Readapt Med Phys. 2006 Jul;49(6):283-8, 370-4.

[206] Debigaré R, Marquis K, Côté CH, Tremblay RR, Michaud A, LeBlanc P, Maltais F. Catabolic/anabolic balance and muscle wasting in patients with COPD. Chest. 2003 Jul;124(1):83-9.

[207] Dyszkiewicz A. Finger cooling test and psychometric analysis in thyroid auxiliary diagnostics. Acta Bioeng Biomech. 2007;9(2):61-8.

[208] Olsen, N; Nielsen, LS. Prevalence of primary Raynaud phenomena in young females. Scandinavian Journal of Clinical and Laboratory Investigation, Volume 38, Issue 8 December 1978 , pages 761 - 764.

[209] Garrison RL, Breeding PC. A metabolic basis for fibromyalgia and its related disorders: the possible role of resistance to thyroid hormone. Med Hypotheses. 2003 Aug;61(2):182-9.

[210] Hayashi M, Shimohira M, Saisho S, Shimozawa K, Iwakawa Y. Sleep disturbance in children with growth hormone deficiency. Brain Dev. 1992 May;14(3):170-4.

[211] Guilhaume A, Benoit O, Gourmelen M, Richardet JM. Relationship between sleep stage IV deficit and reversible HGH deficiency in psychosocial dwarfism. Pediatr Res. 1982 Apr;16(4 Pt 1):299-303.

[212] Guran T, Bircan R, Turan S, Bereket A. Alopecia: association with resistance to thyroid hormones. J Pediatr Endocrinol Metab. 2009 Nov;22(11):1075-81.

[213] Kramer CK, von Mühlen D, Kritz-Silverstein D, Barrett-Connor E. Treated hypothyroidism, cognitive function, and depressed mood in old age: the Rancho Bernardo Study. Eur J Endocrinol. 2009 Dec;161(6):917-21.

[214] Veras AB, Nardi AE. The complex relationship between hypogonadism and major depression in a young male. Prog Neuropsychopharmacol Biol Psychiatry. 2010 Mar 17;34(2):421-2.

[215] Sarrel PM. Psychosexual effects of menopause: role of androgens. Am J Obstet Gynecol. 1999 Mar;180(3 Pt 2):S319-24.

[216] Söderpalma AHV, Lindseya S, et al. Administration of progesterone produces mild sedative-like effects in men and women. Psychoneuroendocrinology, Volume 29, Issue 3, April 2004, Pages 339-354.

[217] Kelly DF, McArthur DL, Levin H, Swimmer S, Dusick JR, Cohan P, Wang C, Swerdloff R. Neurobehavioral and quality of life changes associated with growth hormone insufficiency after complicated mild, moderate, or severe traumatic brain injury. J Neurotrauma. 2006 Jun;23(6):928-42.

[218] Thomsen AF, Kvist TK, Andersen PK, Kessing LV. The risk of affective disorders in patients with adrenocortical insufficiency. Psychoneuroendocrinology. 2006 Jun;31(5):614-22.

[219] Bhagia V, Gilkison C, et al. Effect of recombinant growth hormone replacement in a growth hormone deficient subject recovering from mild traumatic brain injury: A case report. Brain Inj. 2010;24(3):560-7.

[220] Waters DL, Qualls CR, Dorin RI, Veldhuis JD, Baumgartner RN. Altered growth hormone, cortisol, and leptin secretion in healthy elderly persons with sarcopenia and mixed body composition phenotypes. J Gerontol A Biol Sci Med Sci. 2008 May;63(5):536-41.

[221] Roubenoff R, Rall LC, Veldhuis JD, Kehayias JJ, Rosen C, Nicolson M, Lundgren N, Reichlin S. The relationship between growth hormone kinetics and sarcopenia in postmenopausal women: the role of fat mass and leptin. J Clin Endocrinol Metab. 1998 May;83(5):1502-6.

[222] Park YJ, Yoon JW, et al. Subclinical hypothyroidism might increase the risk of transient atrial fibrillation after coronary artery bypass grafting. Ann Thorac Surg. 2009 Jun;87(6):1846-52.

[223] Leong KS, Mann P, et al. The influence of growth hormone replacement on heart rate variability in adults with growth hormone deficiency. Clin Endocrinol (Oxf). 2001 Jun;54(6):819-26.

[224] Erfurth EM, Bülow B, Eskilsson J, Hagmar L. High incidence of cardiovascular disease and increased prevalence of cardiovascular risk factors in women with hypopituitarism not receiving growth hormone treatment: preliminary results. Growth Horm IGF Res. 1999 Apr;9 Suppl A:21-4.

Program 120® Team

[225] Lioté F, Orcel P. Osteoarticular disorders of endocrine origin. Baillieres Best Pract Res Clin Rheumatol. 2000 Jun;14(2):251-76.
[226] Tauchmanova L, Di Somma C, et al. The role for growth hormone in linking arthritis, osteoporosis, and body composition. J Endocrinol Invest. 2007;30(6 Suppl):35-41.
[227] Wüster C, Härle U, et al. Benefits of growth hormone treatment on bone metabolism, bone density and bone strength in growth hormone deficiency and osteoporosis. Growth Horm IGF Res. 1998 Feb;8 Suppl A:87-94.
[228] Kapila S, Wang W, Uston K. Matrix metalloproteinase induction by relaxin causes cartilage matrix degradation in target synovial joints. Ann N Y Acad Sci. 2009 Apr;1160:322-8.
[229] Cole JA, Rothman KJ, Cabral HJ, Zhang Y, Farraye FA. Migraine, fibromyalgia, and depression among people with IBS: a prevalence study. BMC Gastroenterol. 2006 Sep 28;6:26.
[230] Riedl A, Schmidtmann M, et al. Somatic comorbidities of irritable bowel syndrome: a systematic analysis. J Psychosom Res. 2008 Jun;64(6):573-82.
[231] Spaziani R, Bayati A, et al. Vagal dysfunction in irritable bowel syndrome assessed by rectal distension and baroreceptor sensitivity. Neurogastroenterol Motil. 2008 Apr;20(4):336-42.
[232] Phillips AD, Smith MW, Walker-Smith JA. Selective alteration of brush-border hydrolases in intestinal diseases in childhood. Clin Sci (Lond). 1988 Feb;74(2):193-200.
[233] Riedl A, Schmidtmann M, et al. Somatic comorbidities of irritable bowel syndrome: a systematic analysis. J Psychosom Res. 2008 Jun;64(6):573-82.
[234] Krishna AY, Blevins LS Jr. Case report: reversible gastroparesis in patients with hypopituitary disease. Am J Med Sci. 1996 Jul;312(1):43-5.
[235] Hansen GH, Niels-Christiansen LL, Immerdal L, Danielsen EM. Antibodies in the small intestine: mucosal synthesis and deposition of anti-glycosyl IgA, IgM, and IgG in the enterocyte brush border. Am J Physiol Gastrointest Liver Physiol. 2006 Jul;291(1):G82-90.

[236] Bates SL, Sharkey KA, Meddings JB. Vagal involvement in dietary regulation of nutrient transport. Am J Physiol. 1998 Mar;274(3 Pt 1):G552-60.

[237] Kozakova H, Kolinska J, et al. Effect of bacterial monoassociation on brush-border enzyme activities in ex-germ-free piglets: comparison of commensal and pathogenic Escherichia coli strains. Microbes Infect. 2006 Sep;8(11):2629-39.

[238] Kuś E, Karowicz-Bilińska A. The influence of steroid sex hormones on collagen composition in post-operative wounds after long-term treatment with anticoagulants. Ginekol Pol. 2009 Nov;80(11):814-8.

[239] Berga SL, Loucks TL. The diagnosis and treatment of stress-induced anovulation. Minerva Ginecol. 2005 Feb;57(1):45-54.

[240] Tscherne G. [Hormonal disorders, menstrual irregularities and future fertility] [Article in German] Gynakol Geburtshilfliche Rundsch. 2003 Jun;43(3):152-7.

[241] Chelimsky G, Madan S, et al. A comparison of dysautonomias comorbid with cyclic vomiting syndrome and with migraine. Gastroenterol Res Pract. 2009;2009:701019.

[242] Scher AI, Launer LJ. Migraine: migraine with aura increases the risk of stroke. Nat Rev Neurol. 2010 Mar;6(3):128-9.

[243] Saarikoski S, Yliskoski M, Penttilä I. Sequential use of norethisterone and natural progesterone in pre-menopausal bleeding disorders. Maturitas. 1990 Jun;12(2):89-97.

[244] Ustinova EE, Fraser MO, Pezzone MA. Cross-talk and sensitization of bladder afferent nerves. Neurourol Urodyn. 2010;29(1):77-81.

[245] de Groat WC, Yoshimura N. Afferent nerve regulation of bladder function in health and disease. Handb Exp Pharmacol. 2009;(194):91-138.

[246] From http://kidney.niddk.nih.gov/kudiseases/pubs/interstitialcystitis/ .Accessed 2010 March 20.

[247] Rev Urol. 2002; 4(Suppl 1): S3–S8.

[248] Schmidtova E, Kelemenova S, Ostatnikova D. Testosterone supplementation therapy as a treatment of hypogonadism. Bratisl Lek Listy. 2009;110(12):765-72.

[249] Janssen YJ, Doornbos J, Roelfsema F. Changes in muscle volume, strength, and bioenergetics during recombinant human growth hormone (GH) therapy in adults with GH deficiency. J Clin Endocrinol Metab. 1999 Jan;84(1):279-84.

[250] Burk CJ, Ciocca G, Heath CR, Duarte A, Dohil M, Connelly EA. Addison's disease, diffuse skin, and mucosal hyperpigmenation with subtle "flu-like" symptoms--a report of two cases. Pediatr Dermatol. 2008 Mar-Apr;25(2):215-8.

[251] Silver RM, Heyes MP, et al. Scleroderma, fasciitis, and eosinophilia associated with the ingestion of tryptophan. N Engl J Med. 1990 Mar 29;322(13):874-81.

[252] Liptan GL. Fascia: A missing link in our understanding of the pathology of fibromyalgia. J Bodyw Mov Ther. 2010 Jan;14(1):3-12.

[253] Melham TJ, Sevier TL, Malnofski MJ, Wilson JK, Helfst RH. Chronic ankle pain and fibrosis successfully treated with a new non-invasive augmented soft tissue mobilization (ASTM): A case report. Medicine and Science in Sports and Exercise. 1998; 30(6): 801-804.

[254] Chakrabarty S, Zoorob R. Fibromyalgia. Am Fam Physician. 2007 Jul 15;76(2):247-54.

[255] Ge HY, Nie H, et al. Contribution of the local and referred pain from active myofascial trigger points in fibromyalgia syndrome. Pain. 2009 Dec 15;147(1-3):233-40.

[256] Smith KJ, McDonald WI. Spontaneous and mechanically evoked activity due to central demyelinating lesion. Nature. 1980 Jul 10;286(5769):154-5.

[257] Melmed S. Acromegaly and cancer: not a problem? J Clin Endocrinol Metab. 2001 Jul;86(7):2929-34.

[258] Kuijpens JL, Nyklíctek I, et al. Hypothyroidism might be related to breast cancer in post-menopausal women. Thyroid. 2005 Nov;15(11):1253-9.

[259] Campagnoli C, Abba C, Ambroggio S, Peris C. Pregnancy, progesterone and progestins in relation to breast cancer risk. J Steroid Biochem Mol Biol. 2005 Dec;97(5):441-50.

[260] Li CI, Mathes RW, et al. Migraine history and breast cancer risk among postmenopausal women. J Clin Oncol. 2010 Feb 20;28(6):1005-10.

[261] Maes M, Mihaylova I, et al. Increased plasma peroxides and serum oxidized low density lipoprotein antibodies in major depression: Markers that further explain the higher incidence of neurodegeneration and coronary artery disease. J Affect Disord. 2010 Jan 16.

[262] From www.merriam-webster.com/dictionary/paresthesia. Accessed 2010 Mar 22.

[263] Ramachandran TS, Sater RA. Acute Inflammatory Demyelinating Polyradiculoneuropathy.   Online   at http://emedicine.medscape.com/article/1169959-print. Accessed 2010 March 22.

[264] Erdem U, Ozdegirmenci O, et al. Dry eye in post-menopausal women using hormone replacement therapy. Maturitas. 2007 Mar 20;56(3):257-62.

[265] Psaty, BM, Smith NL, et al. Hormone Replacement Therapy, Prothrombotic Mutations, and the Risk of Incident Nonfatal Myocardial Infarction in Postmenopausal Women. JAMA. 2001;285:906-913.

[266] Kuś E, Karowicz-Bilińska A. The influence of steroid sex hormones on collagen composition in post-operative wounds after long-term treatment with anticoagulants. Ginekol Pol. 2009 Nov;80(11):814-8.

[267] Bidlingmaier M, Strasburger CJ. Growth hormone. Handb Exp Pharmacol. 2010;(195):187-200.

[268] Koelling S, Miosge N. Gender differences of chondrogenic progenitor cells in late stages of osteoarthritis. Arthritis Rheum. 2010 Jan 13.

[269] Nishioka T, Kurokawa H, et al. Differential changes of corticotropin releasing hormone (CRH) concentrations in plasma and synovial fluids of patients with rheumatoid arthritis (RA). Endocr J. 1996 Apr;43(2):241-7.

[270] Obtained from www.foodallergytest.com/fibromyalgia.html. Access 2010 March 22.

[271] [no author listed] C-Reactive Protein. [online] Available at www.nlm.nih.gov/medlineplus/ency/article/003356.htm. Accessed 2006 Sep 1.

[272] [no author listed] hs-CRP. [online] Available at www.labtestsonline.org/understanding/analytes/hscrp/test.html. Accessed 2006 Sep 1.

[273] [no author listed] C-Reactive Protein. [online] Available at www.nlm.nih.gov/medlineplus/ency/article/003356.htm. Accessed 2006 Sep 1.

[274] Brigden ML. Clinical utility of the erythrocyte sedimentation rate. Am Fam Physician. 1999 Oct 1;60(5):1443-50.

[275] Fauchald P, Rygvold O, Oystese B. Temporal arteritis and polymyalgia rheumatica: clinical and biopsy findings. Ann Intern Med 1972;77:845-52.

[276] May HT, Alharethi R, Anderson JL, Muhlestein JB, Reyna SP, Bair TL, Horne BD, Kfoury AG, Carlquist JF, Renlund DG. Homocysteine Levels Are Associated with Increased Risk of Congestive Heart Failure in Patients with and without Coronary Artery Disease. Cardiology. 2006 Aug 28;107(3):178-184.

[277] Rauramaa R, Vaisanen S, Mercuri M, Rankinen T, Penttila I, Bond MG.
Association of risk factors and body iron status to carotid atherosclerosis in middle-aged eastern Finnish men. Eur Heart J. 1994 Aug;15(8):1020-7.

[278] Berglund M, Lind B, Bjornberg KA, Palm B, Einarsson O, Vahter M. Inter-individual variations of human mercury exposure biomarkers: a cross-sectional assessment. Environ Health. 2005 Oct 3;4:20.

[279] Muran PJ. Mercury elimination with oral DMPS, DMSA, vitamin C, and glutathione: an observational clinical review. Altern Ther Health Med. 2006 May-Jun;12(3):70-5.

[280] Dargan,PI; Giles, LJ; et al. Case Report: Severe Mercuric Sulphate Poisoning Treated With 2,3-Dimercaptopropane-1-Sulphonate and Haemodiafiltration. Crit Care 7(3), 2003. © 2003 BioMed Central, Ltd.

[281][no author listed] Triglyceride level. [online] Available at www.nlm.nih.gov/medlineplus/ency/article/003493.htm. Accessed 2006 Sep 1.

[282] [no author listed] Triglyceride level. [online] Available at www.nlm.nih.gov/medlineplus/ency/article/003493.htm. Accessed 2006 Sep 1.

[283]Borm K, Slawik M, Beuschlein F, Seiler L, Flohr F, Berg A, Koenig A, Reincke M. Low-dose glucose infusion after achieving critical hypoglycemia during insulin tolerance testing: effects on time of hypoglycemia, neuroendocrine stress response and patient's discomfort in a pilot study. Eur J Endocrinol. 2005 Oct;153(4):521-6.

[284]Murray, R.D. & Shalet, S.M. (2001) Insulin sensitivity is impaired in adults with both severe GH deficiency and GH insufficiency. 83rd Annual Meeting of the Endocrine Society, OR57-3, 145.

[285]Francisco, G., Hernández, C., Galard, R., Simó. R. Usefulness of Homeostasis Model Assessment for Identifying Subjects at Risk for Hypoglycemia Failure during the Insulin Hypoglycemia Test, The Journal of Clinical Endocrinology & Metabolism Vol. 89, No. 7 3408-3412. Copyright © 2004 by The Endocrine Society.

[286]Francisco, G., Hernández, C., Galard, R., Simó. R. Usefulness of Homeostasis Model Assessment for Identifying Subjects at Risk for Hypoglycemia Failure during the Insulin Hypoglycemia Test, The Journal of Clinical Endocrinology & Metabolism Vol. 89, No. 7 3408-3412. Copyright © 2004 by The Endocrine Society.

[287]Tsagarakis S, Vassiliadi D, Thalassinos N. Endogenous subclinical hypercortisolism: Diagnostic uncertainties and clinical implications. J Endocrinol Invest. 2006 May;29(5):471-82.

[288]Burger, HG. Diagnostic role of follicle-stimulating hormone (FSH) measurements during the menopausal transition--an analysis of FSH, oestradiol and inhibin. Eur J Endocrinol 1994 Jan;130(1):38-42.

[289][no author listed] Sex hormone binding globulin. From Wikipedia, the free encyclopedia.. [online] Available at en.wikipedia.org/wiki/Sex_hormone_binding_globulin. Accessed 2006 Sep 3.

[290] Winters, S.J. Chapter 4 - LABORATORY ASSESSMENT OF TESTICULAR FUNCTION, August 17, 2004. [online] Available at www.endotext.org/male/male4/male4.htm. Accessed 2006 Sep 3.

[291] Saxena T, Maheshwari S, Goyal RK. Serum insulin assay: an important therapeutic tool in management of freshly diagnosed type 2 diabetes mellitus. J Assoc Physicians India. 2000 Aug;48(8):815-7.

[292] Garber AJ, Moghissi ES,Bransome ED Jr, et al. American College of Endocrinology position statement on inpatient diabetes and metabolic control. Endocr Pract. 2004;10(suppl 2): 4-9.

[293] American Diabetes Association (ADA). Standards of medical care for patients with diabetes mellitus. Diabetes Care 2003;26(Suppl 1):S33-S50.

[294] United States Department of Health and Human Services. FY 2007 HHS Annual Plan. [online] Available at www.hhs.gov/budget/07plan/sGoal3.html. Accessed 2006 Sep 1.

[295] Neill, R., Speaker: Steven H. Woolf, MD, MPH. Five Steps to Easing Devotion to Glycemic Control. Presented at the The 50th Annual Meeting of the American Academy of Family Physicians Scientific Assembly. [online] Available at www.medscape.com/viewarticle/431920. Accessed 2006 Sep 1.

[296] Breault JL, Goodall CR, Fos PJ. Data mining a diabetic data warehouse. Artif Intell Med. 2002 Sep-Oct;26(1-2):37-54.

[297] El-Kebbi, I.M., Ziemer, D.C., Cook, C.B., Gallina, D.L., Barnes, C.S., Phillips, L.S. Utility of Casual Postprandial Glucose Levels in Type 2 Diabetes Management. Diabetes Care 27:335-339, 2004 © 2004 by the American Diabetes Association, Inc.

[298] Binkley N, Krueger D, Cowgill CS, Plum L, Lake E, Hansen KE, et al. Assay variation confounds the diagnosis of hypovitaminosis D: a call for standardization. J Clin Endocrinol Metab 2004;89:3152-7.

[299] Chandran, M, Phillips, Sa, Ciaraldi, T, Henry, RR. Adiponectin: More Than Just Another Fat Cell Hormone? Diabetes Care 26:2442-2450, 2003. © 2003 by the American Diabetes Association, Inc.

[300] Arita Y, Kihara S, Ouchi N, Takahashi M, Maeda K, Miyagawa J, Hotta K, Shimomura I, Nakamura T, Miyaoka K, Kuriyama H, Nishida M, Yamashita S, Okubo K, Matsubara K, Muraguchi M, Ohmoto Y,

Funahashi T, Matsuzawa Y: Paradoxical decrease of an adipose-specific protein, adiponectin, in obesity. Biochem Biophys Res Commun 257:79–83, 1999.

[301] [no author listed] Overweight and Obesity: Defining Overweight and Obesity. [online] Available at www.cdc.gov/nccdphp/dnpa/obesity/defining.htm. Accessed 2006 Sep 3.

[302] Johnson, TRC; Nikolaou, K; et al. ECG-Gated 64-MDCT Angiography in the Differential Diagnosis of Acute Chest Pain. Am J Roentgenol. 2007;188(1):76-82. ©2007 American Roentgen Ray Society.

[303] Shengxu Li, MD, MPH; Wei Chen, MD, PhD; Sathanur R. Srinivasan, PhD; M. Gene Bond, PhD; Rong Tang, MD, MS; Elaine M. Urbina, MD; Gerald S. Berenson, MD. Childhood Cardiovascular Risk Factors and Carotid Vascular Changes in Adulthood. The Bogalusa Heart Study. JAMA. 2003;290:2271-2276.

[304] Homma, S., Hirose, N., Ishida, H., Ishii, T., Araki, G. Carotid Plaque and Intima-Media Thickness Assessed by B-Mode Ultrasonography in Subjects Ranging From Young Adults to Centenarians. Stroke 2001;32:830.) © 2001 American Heart Association, Inc.

Original Contributions.

[305] Eskes SA, Tomasoa NB, et al. Establishment of reference values for endocrine tests. Part VII: growth hormone deficiency. Neth J Med. 2009 Apr;67(4):127-33.

[306] Found at www.foodallergytest.com/fibromyalgia.html. Accessed 2010 March 22.

[307] Rosano GM, Webb CM, et al. Natural progesterone, but not medroxyprogesterone acetate, enhances the beneficial effect of estrogen on exercise-induced myocardial ischemia in postmenopausal women. J Am Coll Cardiol. 2000 Dec;36(7):2154-9.

[308] McCrohon JA, Nakhla S, Jessup W, Stanley KK, Celermajer DS. Estrogen and progesterone reduce lipid accumulation in human monocyte-derived macrophages: a sex-specific effect. Circulation. 1999 Dec 7;100(23):2319-25.

[309] Gadducci A, Biglia N, Cosio S, Sismondi P, Genazzani AR. Progestagen component in combined hormone replacement therapy in postmenopausal women and breast cancer risk: a debated clinical issue. Gynecol Endocrinol. 2009;25(12):807-15.

[310] Wood CE, Register TC, Lees CJ, Chen H, Kimrey S, Cline JM. Effects of estradiol with micronized progesterone or medroxyprogesterone acetate on risk markers for breast cancer in postmenopausal monkeys. Breast Cancer Res Treat. 2007 Jan;101(2):125-34.

[311] Campagnoli C, Clavel-Chapelon F, Kaaks R, Peris C, Berrino F. Progestins and progesterone in hormone replacement therapy and the risk of breast cancer. J Steroid Biochem Mol Biol. 2005 Jul;96(2):95-108

[312] Fettes I. Migraine in the menopause. Neurology. 1999;53(4 Suppl 1):S29-33.

[313] Author unkown. http://www.lyrica.com/main_how_lyrica_works.aspx. Accessed 2010 March 08.

[314] Streiner DL. Adding zolpidem to CBT produces limited benefits in persistent insomnia. Evid Based Ment Health. 2010 Feb;13(1):28.

[315] Cuddy JS, Reinert AR, Hansen KC, Ruby BC. Effects of modafinil and sleep loss on physiological parameters. Mil Med. 2008 Nov;173(11):1092-7.

[316] Brola W, Ziomek M, Czernicki J. [Fatigue syndrome in chronic neurological disorders] [Article in Polish] Neurol Neurochir Pol. 2007 Jul-Aug;41(4):340-9.

[317] Harbuz M. Neuroendocrinology of autoimmunity. Int Rev Neurobiol. 2002;52:133-61.

[318] Hickey M, Krikun G, Kodaman P, Schatz F, Carati C, Lockwood CJ. Long-term progestin-only contraceptives result in reduced endometrial blood flow and oxidative stress. J Clin Endocrinol Metab. 2006 Sep;91(9):3633-8. Epub 2006 Jun 6.

[319] Bongers MY, Mol BW, Brölmann HA. Current treatment of dysfunctional uterine bleeding. Maturitas. 2004 Mar 15;47(3):159-74.

Real Fibromyalgia Rx – A Pituitary Perspective

[320] Gadducci A, Biglia N, Cosio S, Sismondi P, Genazzani AR. Progestagen component in combined hormone replacement therapy in postmenopausal women and breast cancer risk: a debated clinical issue. Gynecol Endocrinol. 2009;25(12):807-15.

[321] Wood CE, Register TC, Lees CJ, Chen H, Kimrey S, Cline JM. Effects of estradiol with micronized progesterone or medroxyprogesterone acetate on risk markers for breast cancer in postmenopausal monkeys. Breast Cancer Res Treat. 2007 Jan;101(2):125-34.

[322] Blaney GP, Albert PJ, Proal AD. Vitamin D metabolites as clinical markers in autoimmune and chronic disease. Ann N Y Acad Sci. 2009 Sep;1173:384-90.

[323] Cooke GL, Chien A, Brodsky A, Lee RC. Incidence of hypertrophic scars among African Americans linked to vitamin D-3 metabolism? J Natl Med Assoc. 2005 Jul;97(7):1004-9.

[324] Akkuş S, Naziroğlu M, Eriş S, Yalman K, Yilmaz N, Yener M Levels of lipid peroxidation, nitric oxide, and antioxidant vitamins in plasma of patients with fibromyalgia. Cell Biochem Funct. 2009 Jun;27(4):181-5.

[325] Altindag O, Celik H. Total antioxidant capacity and the severity of the pain in patients with fibromyalgia. Redox Rep. 2006;11(3):131-5.

[326] Köhrle J. The deiodinase family: selenoenzymes regulating thyroid hormone availability and action. Cell Mol Life Sci. 2000 Dec;57(13-14):1853-63.

[327] Köhrle J. The deiodinase family: selenoenzymes regulating thyroid hormone availability and action. Cell Mol Life Sci. 2000 Dec;57(13-14):1853-63.

[328] Ko GD, Nowacki NB, Arseneau L, Eitel M, Hum A. Omega-3 fatty acids for neuropathic pain: case series. Clin J Pain. 2010 Feb;26(2):168-72.

[329] Psota TL, Gebauer SK, Kris-Etherton P. Dietary omega-3 fatty acid intake and cardiovascular risk. Am J Cardiol. 2006 Aug 21;98(4A):3i-18i.

[330] Cordero MD, Moreno-Fernández AM, et al. Coenzyme Q10 distribution in blood is altered in patients with fibromyalgia. Clin Biochem. 2009 May;42(7-8):732-5.

[331] Lister RE. An open, pilot study to evaluate the potential benefits of coenzyme Q10 combined with Ginkgo biloba extract in fibromyalgia syndrome. J Int Med Res. 2002 Mar-Apr;30(2):195-9.

[332] Ortancil O, Sanli A, Eryuksel R, Basaran A, Ankarali H. Association between serum ferritin level and fibromyalgia syndrome. Eur J Clin Nutr. 2010 Mar;64(3):308-12.

[333] No author listed. From http://www.youngliving.us/pdfs/PIP_Deep_Relief.pdf. Accessed 2010 April 03.

[334] Méndez JD, Hernández MP. [Article in Spanish] [Effect of L-arginine and polyamines on sperm motility] Ginecol Obstet Mex. 1993 Aug;61:229-34.

[335] Lohiya NK, Manivannan B, Bhande SS, Panneerdoss S, Garg S. Perspectives of contraceptive choices for men. Indian J Exp Biol. 2005 Nov;43(11):1042-7.

[336] Online. No author listed. New male contraceptive found 99 percent effective. http://www.cnn.com/HEALTH/9604/02/nfm/index.html. Accessed 2010 March 26.

[337] Welder AA, Robertson JW, Melchert RB. Toxic effects of anabolic-androgenic steroids in primary rat hepatic cell cultures. J Pharmacol Toxicol Methods. 1995 Aug;33(4):187-95.

[338] Tamimi RM, Hankinson SE, et al. Combined estrogen and testosterone use and risk of breast cancer in postmenopausal women. Arch Intern Med. 2006 Jul 24;166(14):1483-9.

[339] Hargrove JT, Maxson WS, Wentz AC. Absorption of oral progesterone is influenced by vehicle and particle size. Am J Obstet Gynecol. 1989 Oct;161(4):948-51.

[340] Baglietto L, Severi G, et al. Circulating steroid hormone levels and risk of breast cancer for postmenopausal women. Cancer Epidemiol Biomarkers Prev. 2010 Feb;19(2):492-502.

[341] Ruutiainen K. The effect of an oral contraceptive containing ethinylestradiol and desogestrel on hair growth and hormonal

parameters of hirsute women. Int J Gynaecol Obstet. 1986 Oct;24(5):361-8.

[342] Gutierrez, MA; Stimmel, GL. Management of and Counseling for Psychotropic Drug-Induced Sexual Dysfunction. Pharmacotherapy 19(7):823-831, 1999. © 1999 Pharmacotherapy Publications.

[343] Baulieu EE. Dehydroepiandrosterone (DHEA): a fountain of youth? J Clin Endocrinol Metab 1996;81:3147-51.

[344] Regelson W, Loria R, Kalimi M. Hormonal intervention: "buffer hormones" or "state dependency." The role of dehydro-epiandrosterone (DHEA), thyroid hormone, estrogen and hypophysectomy in aging. Ann NY Acad Sci 1988;521:260-73.

[345] Cameron DR, Braunstein GD. The use of dehydroepiandrosterone therapy in clinical practice. Treat Endocrinol. 2005;4(2):95-114.

[346] Cameron DR, Braunstein GD. The use of dehydroepiandrosterone therapy in clinical practice. Treat Endocrinol. 2005;4(2):95-114.

[347] Brown GA, Vukovich M, King DS. Testosterone prohormone supplements. Med Sci Sports Exerc. 2006 Aug;38(8):1451-61

[348] Zdrojewicz Z ; Kesik S.[Dehydroepiandrosterone (DHEA)--youth hormone?]
Wiad Lek. 2001; 54(11-12):693-704 (ISSN: 0043-5147). Available online at www.medsape.com. Accessed 2006 Sep 4.

[349] Furutama D, Fukui R, Amakawa M, Ohsawa N. Inhibition of migration and proliferation of vascular smooth muscle cells by dehydroepiandrosterone sulfate. Biochim Biophys Acta. 1998 Feb 27;1406(1):107-14.

[350] Herrington DM. Dehydroepiandrosterone and coronary atherosclerosis. Ann N Y Acad Sci. 1995 Dec 29;774:271-80.

[351] Barret-Connor E, Knaw KT, Yen SSC. A prospective study of dehydroepiandrosterone sulfate, mortality and cardiovascular disease. N Engl J Med. 1986 Dec 11; 315:1519-24.

[352] Nestler JE. Regulation of human dehydroepiandrosterone metabolism by insulin. Ann NY Acad Sci 1995;774:73-81.

[353] Villareal DT, Holloszy JO. Effect of DHEA on abdominal fat and insulin action in elderly women and men: a randomized controlled trial. JAMA. 2004 Nov 10;292(18):2243-8.

[354] Derksen RH. Dehydroepiandrosterone (DHEA) and systemic lupus erythematosus. Semin Arthritis Rheum. 1998; 27:335-47.
[355] Rabkin JG, Ferrando SJ, Wagner GJ et al. DHEA treatment for HIV+ patients: effects on mood, androgenic and anabolic parameters. Psychoneuroendocrinology. 2000; 25(1):53-68.
[356] Vermeulen A, Kaufman JM, Giagulli VA. Influence of some biological indexes on sex hormone-binding globulin and androgen levels in aging or obese males. J Clin Endocrinol Metab. 1996;81:1821-1826.
[357] Villareal DT. Effects of dehydroepiandrosterone on bone mineral density: what implications for therapy? Treat Endocrinol. 2002;1(6):349-57.
[358] Perrini S ; Laviola L ; Natalicchio A ; Giorgino F. Associated hormonal declines in aging: DHEAS. J Endocrinol Invest. 2005; 28(3 Suppl):85-93 (ISSN: 0391-4097).
[359] Arlt W. Dehydroepiandrosterone replacement therapy. Semin Reprod Med. 2004 Nov;22(4):379-88.
[360] Eser D, Schule C, Baghai TC, Romeo E, Uzunov DP, Rupprecht R. Neuroactive steroids and affective disorders. Pharmacol Biochem Behav. 2006 Jul 8.
[361] Wolkowitz OM, Reus VI, Roberts E, Manfredi F, Chan T, Raum WJ, Ormiston S, Johnson R, Canick J, Brizendine L, Weingartner H. Dehydroepiandrosterone (DHEA) treatment of depression. Biol Psychiatry. 1997 Feb 1;41(3):311-8.
[362] Barrett-Connor, E. (1992) Lower endogenous androgen levels and dyslipidemia in men with non insulin-dependent diabetes mellitus. Annals of Internal Medicine, 117, 807–811.
[363] Villareal DT, Holloszy JO. Effect of DHEA on abdominal fat and insulin action in elderly women and men: a randomized controlled trial. JAMA. 2004 Nov 10;292(18):2243-8.
[364] Hirshman E; Wells E; Wierman ME; Anderson B; Butler A; Senholzi M; Fisher J. The effect of dehydroepiandrosterone (DHEA) on recognition memory decision processes and discrimination in postmenopausal women. Psychon Bull Rev. 2003; 10(1):125-34 (ISSN: 1069-9384).

[365] Brooke AM, Kalingag LA, Miraki-Moud F, Camacho-Hubner C, Maher KT, Walker DM, Hinson JP, Monson JP. Dehydroepiandrosterone (DHEA) improves psychological well-being in male and female hypopituitary patients on maintenance growth hormone replacement. J Clin Endocrinol Metab. 2006 Jul 18.

[366] Williams JR. The effects of dehydroepiandrosterone on carcinogenesis, obesity, the immune system, and aging. Lipids. 2000 Mar;35(3):325-31.

[367] Lahita RG. Dehydroepiandrosterone (DHEA) for serious disease, a possibility? Lupus. 1999; 8:169-70.

[368] Villareal DT. Effects of dehydroepiandrosterone on bone mineral density: what implications for therapy? Treat Endocrinol. 2002;1(6):349-57.

[369] Morales AJ, Haubrich RH, Hwang JY, Asakura H, Yen SS. The Effect of Six Months Treatment With a 100 mg Daily Dose of Dehydroepiandrosterone (DHEA) on Circulating Sex Steroids, Body Composition and Muscle Strength in Age-Advanced Men and Women. Clin Endocrinol (Oxf). 1998;49(4):421-432.

[370] Williams CL, Stancel GM. Estrogens and progestins. In: Hardman JG, Limbird LE, Molinoff PB, Rudden RW, eds. Goodman and Gilman's the Pharmacological Basis for Therapeutics. New York, NY: McGraw-Hill; 1996:1411-1440.

[371] Finckh A, Berner IC, Aubry-Rozier B, So AK. A randomized controlled trial of dehydroepiandrosterone in postmenopausal women with fibromyalgia. J Rheumatol. 2005 Jul;32(7):1336-40.

[372] Stanczyk FZ. Best Pract Res Clin Endocrinol Metab. 2006 Jun;20(2):177-91. Diagnosis of hyperandrogenism: biochemical criteria.

[373] Bauer ME. Stress, glucocorticoids and ageing of the immune system. Stress. 2005; 8(1):69-83 (ISSN: 1025-3890).

[374] van Niekerk JK; Huppert FA; Herbert J. Salivary cortisol and DHEA: association with measures of cognition and well-being in normal older men, and effects of three months of DHEA supplementation. Psychoneuroendocrinology. 2001; 26(6):591-612 (ISSN: 0306-4530).

[375] Barclay, L. Medscape Medical News. Prasterone Helpful in Systemic Lupus Erythematosus. [online] Available at www.medscape.com/viewarticle/488995. Accessed 2006 Sep 4.

[376] Lobo, R. Menopause Management for the Millennium. [online] Available at www.medscape.com/viewprogram/213_pnt. Accessed 2006 Sep 4.

[377] Kehinde EO, Akanji AO, Al-Hunayan A, Memon A, Luqmani Y, Al-Awadi KA, Varghese R, Bashir AA, Daar AS. Do differences in age specific androgenic steroid hormone levels account for differing prostate cancer rates between Arabs and Caucasians? Int J Urol. 2006 Apr;13(4):354-61.

[378] Baglietto L, Severi G, et al. Circulating steroid hormone levels and risk of breast cancer for postmenopausal women. Cancer Epidemiol Biomarkers Prev. 2010 Feb;19(2):492-502.

[379] Cobin, Rh. HRT and Cardiocascular Protection (January 2001 -- Live Event). Medical Crossfire, June 2001; Vol. 3 [6]: 139-40.

[380] Hormone Replacement Therapy, Prothrombotic Mutations, and the Risk of Incident Nonfatal Myocardial Infarction in Postmenopausal Women by Bruce M. Psaty, MD, PhD et al. in JAMA. 2001;285:906-913.

[381] Cuatrecasas G, Riudavets C, Güell MA, Nadal A. Growth hormone as concomitant treatment in severe fibromyalgia associated with low IGF-1 serum levels. A pilot study. BMC Musculoskelet Disord. 2007 Nov 30;8:119.

[382] Wingenfeld K, Heim C, et al. HPA axis reactivity and lymphocyte glucocorticoid sensitivity in fibromyalgia syndrome and chronic pelvic pain. Psychosom Med. 2008 Jan;70(1):65-72.

[383] No author listed. Obtained from http://www.rxlist.com/florinef-drug.htm. Accessed 2010 March 26.

[384] No Author Listed. Obtained from http://www.drugs.com/pro/cortef.html. Accesed 2010 March 26.

[385] Morales AJ, Haubrich RH, Hwang JY, Asakura H, Yen SS. The Effect of Six Months Treatment With a 100 mg Daily Dose of Dehydroepiandrosterone (DHEA) on Circulating Sex Steroids, Body

213

Composition and Muscle Strength in Age-Advanced Men and Women. Clin Endocrinol (Oxf). 1998;49(4):421-432.

[386] Melmed S. Acromegaly and cancer: not a problem? J Clin Endocrinol Metab. 2001 Jul;86(7):2929-34.

[387] Tamimi RM, Hankinson SE, et al. Combined estrogen and testosterone use and risk of breast cancer in postmenopausal women. Arch Intern Med. 2006 Jul 24;166(14):1483-9.

[388] Baglietto L, Severi G, et al. Circulating steroid hormone levels and risk of breast cancer for postmenopausal women. Cancer Epidemiol Biomarkers Prev. 2010 Feb;19(2):492-502.

[389] Regan FM, Williams RM, et al. Treatment with Recombinant Human Insulin-Like Growth Factor (rhIGF)-I/rhIGF Binding Protein-3 Complex Improves Metabolic Control in Subjects with Severe Insulin Resistance. J Clin Endocrinol Metab. 2010 Mar 16.

[390] Meisler, JG. Toward Optimal Health: The Experts Provide a Current Perspective on Perimenopause. J Womens Health 12(7):609-615, 2003. © 2003 Mary Ann Liebert, Inc.

[391] At http://www.law.ua.edu/lawreview/articles/Volume%2060/Issue%204/everest.pdf. Accessed 2010 March 20.